AF352858

Insomnia

Insomnia: Beyond Hyperarousal

Special Issue Editor

Célyne Bastien

MDPI • Basel • Beijing • Wuhan • Barcelona • Belgrade • Manchester • Tokyo • Cluj • Tianjin

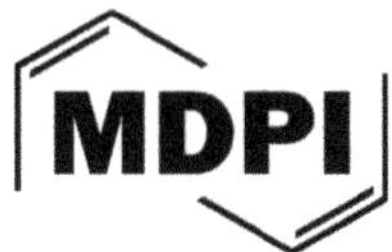

Special Issue Editor
Célyne Bastien
Université Laval
Canada

Editorial Office
MDPI
St. Alban-Anlage 66
4052 Basel, Switzerland

This is a reprint of articles from the Special Issue published online in the open access journal *Brain Sciences* (ISSN 2076-3425) (available at: https://www.mdpi.com/journal/brainsci/special_issues/insomnia_hyperarousal).

For citation purposes, cite each article independently as indicated on the article page online and as indicated below:

LastName, A.A.; LastName, B.B.; LastName, C.C. Article Title. *Journal Name* **Year**, *Article Number*, Page Range.

ISBN 978-3-03936-162-5 (Pbk)
ISBN 978-3-03936-163-2 (PDF)

Cover image courtesy of Célyne Bastien.

Contents

About the Special Issue Editor . . . . **vii**

Célyne Bastien
Does Insomnia Exist without Hyperarousal? What Else Can There Be?
Reprinted from: *Brain Sci.* **2020**, *10*, 225, doi:10.3390/brainsci10040225 . . . . **1**

Ivan Vargas, Anna M. Nguyen, Alexandria Muench, Célyne H. Bastien, Jason G. Ellis and Michael L. Perlis
Acute and Chronic Insomnia: What Has Time and/or Hyperarousal Got to Do with It?
Reprinted from: *Brain Sci.* **2020**, *10*, 71, doi:10.3390/brainsci10020071 . . . . **3**

Reuben D. M. Howlett, Kari A. Lustig, Kevin J. MacDonald and Kimberly A. Cote
Hyperarousal Is Associated with Socioemotional Processing in Individuals with Insomnia Symptoms and Good Sleepers
Reprinted from: *Brain Sci.* **2020**, *10*, 112, doi:10.3390/brainsci10020112 . . . . **15**

Celyne H. Bastien, Jason G. Ellis, Amy Athey, Subhajit Chakravorty, Rebecca Robbins, Adam P. Knowlden, Jonathan Charest and Michael A. Grandner
Driving After Drinking Alcohol Associated with Insufficient Sleep and Insomnia among Student Athletes and Non-Athletes
Reprinted from: *Brain Sci.* **2019**, *9*, 46, doi:10.3390/brainsci9020046 . . . . **37**

Yi Zhou and Brian D. Greenwald
Update on Insomnia after Mild Traumatic Brain Injury
Reprinted from: *Brain Sci.* **2018**, *8*, 223, doi:10.3390/brainsci8120223 . . . . **49**

Laith Thamer Al-Ameri, Talib Saddam Mohsin and Ali Tarik Abdul Wahid
Sleep Disorders Following Mild and Moderate Traumatic Brain Injury
Reprinted from: *Brain Sci.* **2019**, *9*, 10, doi:10.3390/brainsci9010010 . . . . **69**

Alexander Sweetman, Leon Lack and Célyne Bastien
Co-Morbid Insomnia and Sleep Apnea (COMISA): Prevalence, Consequences, Methodological Considerations, and Recent Randomized Controlled Trials
Reprinted from: *Brain Sci.* **2019**, *9*, 371, doi:10.3390/brainsci9120371 . . . . **75**

Cigdem Sahbaz, Ahmet Elbay, Mine Ozcelik and Hakan Ozdemir
Insomnia Might Influence the Thickness of Choroid, Retinal Nerve Fiber and Inner Plexiform Layer
Reprinted from: *Brain Sci.* **2020**, *10*, 178, doi:10.3390/brainsci10030178 . . . . **93**

About the Special Issue Editor

Célyne Bastien, Ph.D., holds bachelor (1989) and Ph.D. (1993) degrees from the University of Ottawa and is currently a full Professor with the School of Psychology at the Université Laval, Québec City, Canada. She is also an active sleep researcher with CERVO. Dr. Bastien is the current President of the Canadian Sleep Society and an active partner of the public campaign on sleep sleeponitcanada.ca (dormezladessuscanada.ca).

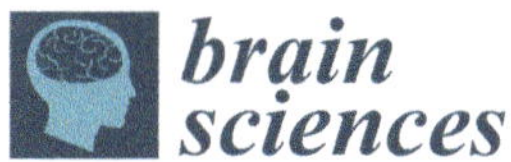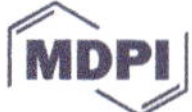

Editorial

Does Insomnia Exist without Hyperarousal? What Else Can There Be?

Célyne Bastien

School of psychology, Laval University, Quebec, QC G1V0A6, Canada; celyne.bastien@psy.ulaval.ca

Received: 7 April 2020; Accepted: 9 April 2020; Published: 10 April 2020

While in ancient Greece, incubation rooms were dedicated to the interpretation of dreams, sleep was also studied by famous philosophers such as Aristotle. In 350 B.C.E., he wrote an essay titled "On Sleep and Sleepiness". In the essay, he described some basics of how sleep was regulated and how it was naturally induced. Nowadays, we know much more about sleep and its regulation (circadian rhythms, homeostatic processes, etc.) and the diurnal consequences of the lack of sleep (poor memory and decision-making, lack of attention, increased car accidents, health issues, etc.).

Although some of us might decide today to cut down on our sleep because of work, family or other related reasons, this choice is voluntary. Involuntary sleep reduction, as it is the case with insomnia, brings its own consequences. With the advent of the modern world and the appearance of stress, we have seen cases of insomnia grow from one century to the other. Today, worldwide, rates of chronic insomnia are nearing 12% of the population, while about 30% of individuals report suffering from an occasional bad night of sleep. Although we know that insomnia, albeit acute or chronic, is often precipitated by an event, one can be predisposed to suffer from it (for example, being a woman or an elderly) and can also maintain sleep difficulties with bad habits (for example, staying in bed while unable to fall asleep).

At the core of insomnia, hyperarousal (cortical and physical) has been recognized as having a dominant role to play. One can be predisposed to have a higher hyperarousal level, or hyperarousal can develop with time. In fact, hyperarousal may be what prevents you from falling asleep and wakes you up during the night, and is reflected through heightened cortical activity, for example. However, hyperarousal might not explain everything. In fact, one perspective offered by Vargas and al. [1] questions if hyperarousal has anything to do with either acute or chronic insomnia. By disentangling how the flight-or-fight response suggested for acute insomnia is different to the learned hyperarousal observed in chronic insomnia, this review sets the tone for the rest of the issue. However, a very innovative way to study arousal, and especially hyperarousal, while looking at socioemotional processing is described by Howlett and colleagues [2]. By studying responses in categorization of face-emotion stimuli and intensity of risk-taking in both good sleepers and individuals suffering of insomnia, these authors suggests that beta activity (which is considered the cortical signature of hyperarousal) interferes differentially in the two studied groups and is not the hallmark of insomnia only.

Two other reviews in the issue discuss different issues. The first one discusses how important and high the rate of comorbid insomnia and apnea is. According to authors [3], insomnia was long considered secondary to apnea, and it is only recently that clinicians have begun to study how these two sleep disorders can be dealt differently treatment wise and explain why response rate was often so low in both previous sleep disorders in treatment studies. Next, a systematic review informs us about the subtle but very disturbing role insomnia plays in traumatic brain injury patients. It is worth mentioning that insomnia in conjunction with drowsiness will definitely impact on brain injury patients' daily life [4]. Recent research in the area of traumatic brain injury is so active that another paper from this issue studies this very interesting area of research, especially when we know that both insomnia and drowsiness are often underdiagnosed and thus undertreated in these patients, while remaining persistent complaints [5].

One of the aims of the present issue was to demystify some of the less explored concepts, which might, in fact, act as precipitating factors of insomnia, maintain it with an active comorbidity or have health and societal consequences superseding hyperarousal. As such, jumping right in, we know that alcohol interferes with sleep, and its abrupt cessation in regular drinkers can also cause severe insomnia. However, what role does insomnia have in risky behavior when an individual also suffers from insomnia? In fact, student athletes are at a higher risk of driving under the influence of alcohol than non-athlete students and, furthermore, especially if they suffer from insomnia [6].

Finally, the last paper of this issue deals with some physical aspects of our body: choroid, retinal nerve fibers and the inner plexiform layer [7]. Not only were those affected in individuals suffering of insomnia, they were more so as the severity of insomnia increased. This new line of research might pave the way not only for future research on insomnia and tissue degeneration, but also for sleep and its implications together in non-degenerative profiles as measured by optical coherence tomography.

As more research evolves on insomnia treatment and sleep per se, the future is bright for those working in these areas of research. It is not imminent that insomnia rates will dramatically drop, and more research to understand how it develops and is maintained as well as the best way to treat it are still more than ever needed. Let us disseminate our knowledge, to nurture what will need to be done next.

Conflicts of Interest: The author declares no conflict of interest.

References

1. Vargas, I.; Nguyen, A.M.; Muench, A.; Bastien, C.H.; Ellis, J.G.; Perlis, M.L. Acute and Chronic Insomnia: What Has Time and/or Hyperarousal Got to Do with It? *Brain Sci.* **2020**, *10*, 71. [CrossRef] [PubMed]
2. Howlett, R.D.M.; Lustig, K.A.; MacDonald, K.J.; Cote, K.A. Hyperarousal Is Associated with Socioemotional Processing in Individuals with Insomnia Symptoms and Good Sleepers. *Brain Sci.* **2020**, *10*, 112. [CrossRef] [PubMed]
3. Sweetman, A.; Lack, L.; Bastien, C. Co-Morbid Insomnia and Sleep Apnea (COMISA): Prevalence, Consequences, Methodological Considerations, and Recent Randomized Controlled Trials. *Brain Sci.* **2019**, *9*, 371. [CrossRef]
4. Zhou, Y.; Greenwald, B.D. Update on Insomnia after Mild Traumatic Brain Injury. *Brain Sci.* **2018**, *8*, 223. [CrossRef]
5. Al-Ameri, L.T.; Mohsin, T.S.; Abdul Wahid, A.T. Sleep Disorders Following Mild and Moderate Traumatic Brain Injury. *Brain Sci.* **2019**, *9*, 10. [CrossRef] [PubMed]
6. Bastien, C.H.; Ellis, J.G.; Athey, A.; Chakravorty, S.; Robbins, R.; Knowlden, A.P.; Charest, J.; Grandner, M.A. Driving After Drinking Alcohol Associated with Insufficient Sleep and Insomnia among Student Athletes and Non-Athletes. *Brain Sci.* **2019**, *9*, 46. [CrossRef] [PubMed]
7. Sahbaz, C.; Elbay, A.; Ozcelik, M.; Ozdemir, H. Insomnia Might Influence the Thickness of Choroid, Retinal Nerve Fiber and Inner Plexiform Layer. *Brain Sci.* **2020**, *10*, 178. [CrossRef] [PubMed]

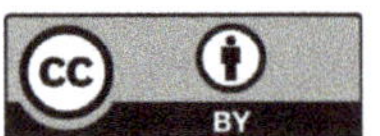

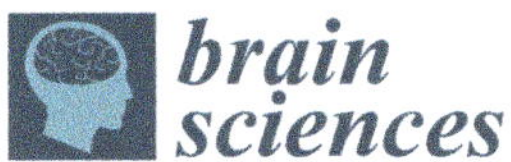 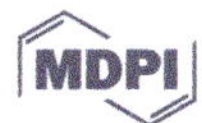

Perspective

Acute and Chronic Insomnia: What Has Time and/or Hyperarousal Got to Do with It?

Ivan Vargas [1,*], Anna M. Nguyen [1], Alexandria Muench [2], Célyne H. Bastien [3], Jason G. Ellis [4] and Michael L. Perlis [2]

1   Department of Psychological Science, University of Arkansas, Fayetteville, AR 72701, USA; atn010@uark.edu
2   Department of Psychiatry, University of Pennsylvania, Philadelphia, PA 19104, USA; amuench@pennmedicine.upenn.edu (A.M.N.); mperlis@upenn.edu (M.L.P.)
3   School of Psychology, Laval University, Quebec, QC G1V 0A6, Canada; celyne.bastien@psy.ulaval.ca
4   Northumbria Center for Sleep Research, Northumbria University, Newcastle NE7 7XA, UK; jason.ellis@northumbria.ac.uk
*   Correspondence: ivvargas@uark.edu; Tel.: +1-479-575-7610

Received: 19 December 2019; Accepted: 25 January 2020; Published: 29 January 2020

Abstract: Nearly one-third of the population reports new onset or acute insomnia in a given year. Similarly, it is estimated that approximately 10% of the population endorses sleep initiation and maintenance problems consistent with diagnostic criteria for chronic insomnia. For decades, acute and chronic insomnia have been considered variations of the same condition or disorder, only really differentiated in terms of chronicity of symptoms (days/weeks versus months). Whether or not acute and chronic insomnia are part of the same phenomena is an important question, one that has yet to be empirically evaluated. The goal of the present theoretical review was to summarize the definitions of acute and chronic insomnia and discuss the role that hyperarousal may have in explaining how the pathophysiology of acute and chronic insomnia is likely different (i.e., what biopsychological factors precipitate and/or perpetuate acute insomnia, chronic insomnia, or both?).

Keywords: insomnia; hyperarousal; diagnostic criteria

---

1. Introduction

There are two general, but fundamental beliefs about insomnia that are critically evaluated in this article: (1) Acute insomnia is simply a briefer form of chronic insomnia, and (2) insomnia (regardless of its chronicity) is characterized by a state of hyperarousal. In order to address these issues, the definitions of, and concepts related to, acute and chronic insomnia and hyperarousal are briefly reviewed. Ultimately, it is argued that the distinction between acute and chronic insomnia needs to be the subject of empirical investigation, especially when evaluating the role of hyperarousal in the pathophysiology of insomnia.

2. Defining Acute and Chronic Insomnia (Just a Matter of Time?)

Acute Insomnia. Historically, acute insomnia (AI) has not been well defined or precisely delineated in the literature, despite its having been included in multiple classification systems since at least the late 1970s [1,2]. Part of the problem is multiple terms have been used to refer to AI over this time frame. AI has been classified as adjustment insomnia, stress-related insomnia, transient psychophysiological insomnia, symptomatic insomnia, sub-acute insomnia, and sub-chronic insomnia [3–10]. Such variability in terminology has discouraged consensus building, both conceptually and operationally. Another problem has been that the durational criteria for AI has been defined by default; by any time period shorter than the criteria for chronic insomnia (CI). Over the years, CI has been variably defined as more than 1 month [11], 3 months [12], or 6 months [3], and therefore,

AI has also been variably defined as shorter than each of these duration thresholds. Still yet another problem, one that also extends to CI, is that AI has not been defined based on quantitative criteria for sleep continuity disturbance (illness severity viz. sleep latency, wake after sleep onset, early morning awakenings, etc.). Finally, it should be noted that the various definitions and nosological classifications for both AI and CI have been made on the basis of consensus opinion and not based on any empirical derivation (e.g., how many consecutive nights must occur until it is unlikely that the insomnia will remit?).

In recent years, the issue of "what is acute insomnia and how should it be defined?" has been the subject of renewed interest, largely owing to the conduct of several natural history studies [10,13,14] and the publication of one theoretical review dedicated to AI [6]. In the review, three definitions of AI (Diagnostic and Statistical Manual of Mental Disorders [DSM], International Classification of Sleep Disorders [ICSD], and International Classification of Diseases [ICD]) were compared and contrasted. The central role of precipitating factors for AI was highlighted. Life stress was identified as a/the primary precipitant for insomnia based on a review of several etiological models, and a formal definition of AI was proffered. The definition had both qualitative and quantitative criteria, included the delineation of sub-states, and required that a precipitating life event or stress condition be identified. The specific definition put forward was as follows: AI is defined as sleep continuity disturbance (i.e., difficulty initiating and/or maintaining sleep) occurring on at least 3 days per week for anywhere between 1 week and 3 months. The more than or equal to one week duration threshold (3-day minimum) allowed for the likely possibility of non-pathologic insomnia (i.e., insomnia as a normal variation in sleep continuity, presumably occurring in association with less than optimal circumstances for sleep [sleep without adequate homeostatic priming or sleep that occurs at times outside the individual's preferred sleep phase]). The remaining time frame (>1 week to 3 months) was subdivided into: Acute (>3–14 days), transient (2–4 weeks), and sub-chronic insomnia (1–3 months). It is important to note that this categorization was not empirically based on insomnia but was in line with other mood disorders [6,12,15]. The quantitative criteria applied to the definition of AI were those that are typically adopted for clinical research [13,16]. This rule is generally applied to typical or average sleep latency and/or wake after sleep onset values. More specifically, individuals that take ≥ 30 minutes to fall asleep or who are awake for periods of this magnitude during the night are identified as having 'difficulty initiating and/or maintaining sleep' (insomnia of a severity that warrants and/or can be successfully treated). While Ellis and colleagues do not, it is also possible to apply the 30-minute rule to early morning awakenings (awakening 30 or more minutes prior to one's desired time to awake is deemed problematic). In addition to chronicity, frequency, and severity criteria, it was also stipulated that an AI episode must have a clear precipitant, i.e., that the individual must be able to identify a triggering event characterized as, "(1) any life event or train of life events that results in a significant reduction in quality of life from the individual's ideal and/or (2) distress at one's current situation" [6]. The concept that AI must be triggered by an event (a bio-behavioral reaction to stress [perceived or real threat]) is further amplified in the closing section of the review. Here Ellis and colleagues suggest that AI may be conceptualized as part of a larger, and non-pathological, biopsychosocial process. That is, acute insomnia may be considered a normal part of the fight/flight response. Evolutionarily speaking, AI likely represents a necessary override to the normal two process regulation of sleep [17]. That is, if it is not safe to sleep, one should not sleep (regardless of the duration of prior wakefulness and/or time of day). This concept is not new but was presaged by Spielman and Glovinsky in the 1990s when they stated, "No matter how important sleep may be, it was adaptively deferred when the mountain lion entered the cave" [7].

Chronic Insomnia. In contrast to AI, the literature on chronic insomnia is extensive [18,19]. As would be expected, formal definitions have been developed and adopted, though not without revisions over the last 40 years. Historically (and as noted above), the definition of what constitutes "chronic" has varied greatly. Presently, CI is a diagnostic category within all three of the major nosological systems: ICSD-3 (Chronic Insomnia Disorder [20]), ICD-11 (Chronic Insomnia [21]) and

DSM-5 (Insomnia Disorder [12]). All three classification systems include as criteria that the sleep problem is: (1) Characterized by difficulty initiating and/or maintaining sleep; (2) associated with significant daytime consequences, impairment, or distress; and (3) present despite adequate opportunity for sleep. The ICSD-3 and the DSM-5 additionally specify that the sleep continuity problem must occur with a frequency ≥ to 3 days per week and be of a duration of at least 3 months. The ICD-11 does not specify quantitative criteria for insomnia frequency or chronicity and none of the diagnostic systems utilize a quantitative threshold for severity (i.e., adopt the 30-minute rule that is commonly used for clinical research [13,16]).

The changes in diagnostic criteria, especially with respect to chronicity, have made it difficult to differentiate what constitutes AI versus CI (i.e., when does AI end and CI begin?). Assuming that AI and CI represent different stages of a single disease process, it may be that the common dichotomization is too simplistic and does not adequately capture the clinical course of insomnia disorder. For example, when conducting a natural history study, we observed that not all individuals experiencing AI go on to recover normal sleep or develop CI, some individuals develop a form of persistent poor sleep that does not meet criteria for either AI or CI [14]. This observation has prompted some investigators to denote a third type of insomnia as "subsyndromal insomnia", "intermediate insomnia", or "persistent poor sleep" [9,13,14,22]. Finally, it should be noted that AI and CI may not represent different stages of a single disease process; it may be that AI and CI are symptomatically similar but are distinct clinical phenomena (e.g., occur with different frequencies and severities) with distinctly different biological bases. For example, acute insomnia may occur in association with hypercortisolemia [23], while chronic insomnia may occur in association with hyperorexinemia [24] or abnormally low levels of γ-aminobutyric acid (GABA) [25].

3. Prevalence and Incidence of Acute and Chronic Insomnia

A number of epidemiological studies have been conducted over the course of the last 30 years [26–28]. Nearly all of these investigations have focused on the prevalence rate of chronic insomnia. In general, chronic insomnia has been found to occur in 6–10% of the population [26–29]. Prevalence rates as high as 30% have been reported when: Duration of illness is not taken into account, qualitative criteria are used for insomnia frequency, and/or when daytime impairment criteria are not used to define "caseness" [27,28]. Data on the prevalence of AI has only recently been published [13]. Using the same criteria as outlined in the previous section, the prevalence rates of AI were 9.5% (USA sample) and 7.9% (UK sample). Alternatively, several studies have attempted to estimate the incidence of acute insomnia (typically defined as new onset insomnia). The first such study was undertaken by Ford and Kamerow (1989) [26]. They reported that the incidence rate of new-onset insomnia was 6.2% [26]. A decade later, a similar study was undertaken by Foley and colleagues [30]. They reported that the three-year incidence rate of insomnia was 15% (or an annual incidence rate of approximately 5%). More recent studies provide convergent data suggesting that the annual incidence of insomnia is between 7–8% for insomnia "syndrome" and up to 30% for the occurrence of "insomnia symptoms" [10,31]. The only study to explicitly assess AI (using diagnostic criteria) reported that the incidence rate of AI was between 31–37% (depending on whether DSM criteria with or without additional case criteria (sleep latency or wake after sleep onset of 30 min or longer and a self-reported increase in daytime impairment) was used) [13].

While there is a large measure of consistency among the AI studies (despite different methods, measures, sampling rates, and time frames), the reported incident rates, for most of these studies, were not truly the incidence of acute insomnia but rather the identification of new onset insomnia of any duration (includes both AI and CI). Put differently, most of the incidence studies used interval assessment strategies, where sleep continuity was profiled every one to three months [10,30,31]. This sampling rate lacks the temporal resolution needed to identify the onset and offset of short bouts of insomnia. In order to resolve such a phenomenon, one would need to start with a proband of good sleepers and assess them on a daily or weekly basis. Our group recently undertook such a study [14].

Using these data, it was determined that the annual incidence of AI was 27% and that the annual incidence rate of CI was 1.8%. Of those that developed AI, approximately 72% went on to recover good sleep and 19% developed persistently poor sleep (i.e., these subjects did not recover good sleep but also did not meet duration and/or severity thresholds consistent with DSM-5 Insomnia Disorder).

In sum, the population prevalence of chronic insomnia is around 10% while up to 30% of the population experiences new onset or acute insomnia on an annual basis. Of those that experience AI, the majority recover, a small minority develop CI, and up to 20% develop an intermediate form of sleep continuity disturbance that does not meet criteria for either AI or CI. The existence of this third group speaks to the need to think more dimensionally about insomnia chronicity and/or the need to create a more pluralistic typology. While this may be done on theoretical grounds, empirically defining what constitutes normal sleeplessness, acute insomnia, persistent poor sleep, and chronic insomnia (and how these stages differ with respect to symptom severity and frequency) will no doubt make clearer how these stages differ with respect to their etiology and pathophysiology.

4. Defining "Hyperarousal"

When acute, hyperarousal occurs as a triggered psychosomatic response to threat-related stimuli. This response, also known as the "fight-or-flight response", is characterized by the activation of the autonomic nervous system and adrenal cortex with corresponding increases in adrenergic and hypothalamic–pituitary–adrenal (HPA) axis activity [32,33]. The physiologic consequences of such activation include increased heart and respiration rate, peripheral vasoconstriction, increased perspiration, dilation of pupils, increased muscle tension, and increased glucose release via the breakdown of glucogenic stores [34–36]. These responses allow the organism to be optimally resourced (for a brief period of time) to fight or flee. While this type of hyperarousal is obviously adaptive, this level of activation is not typically maintained for extended periods of time (e.g., the average HPA axis stress response is between 45–60 minutes from start to finish [35,36]). Put differently, most human stress systems in the body are self-regulating, which prohibits them from staying "on" for extended periods of time [37,38]. This being the case, it has been hypothesized that a secondary process or system exists that allows the individual to maintain an elevated state of "preparedness" in response to longer-lasting environmental demands, if not overt threats [39–41]. This form of "hyperarousal" may consist of a lower-level tonic activation of the fight/flight system [42,43] or the activation of an, as of yet to be identified, alternative system. Consistent with the former point of view, it has been found that individuals who work under chronic stressful circumstances, for example, first responders or military service members, have been shown to exhibit higher levels of HPA and adrenergic activation [44,45], though such activation is of significantly lower magnitude than occurs with fight-or-flight responses [46–48].

5. Hyperarousal in the Context of Insomnia

It is practically axiomatic that insomnia is considered a hyperarousal disorder, i.e., that sleeplessness occurs because of cognitive, and/or somatic, and/or neurophysiologic hyperarousal [49–52]. The evidence base for this belief, however, is not as large or unequivocal as one might expect. In general, the case for hyperarousal is supported by studies of central and/or autonomic nervous systems and endocrine system activation in patients with chronic insomnia as compared to good sleepers. Examples of central nervous system measures include power spectral measures of high frequency electroencephalogram (EEG) activity [51,53,54], EEG-based evoked response potential measures [55,56], imaging measures of brain glucose or oxygen utilization [57], and/or neuroimaging measures of GABA [25,58,59]. Examples of autonomic measures include heart rate [60], heart rate variability [61], electrodermal activity [62], epinephrine or norepinephrine [63], core body temperature measures [64], and/or metabolic rate measures [65]. Endocrine measures typically include blood- and/or saliva-based measures of cortisol [66,67]. It is important to consider, however, that prior research on the hyperarousal theory of insomnia has mostly observed incremental increases in psychobiological indices (e.g., evening levels in cortisol, core body temperature, glucose metabolism, etc.) in comparison to what is "average". For example, while prior studies have shown significantly greater MSLT scores in patients with insomnia (suggesting a greater daytime wake drive relative to controls (i.e., greater hyperarousal)), the mean group differences ranged from 2–5 minutes [68,69]. That is, these studies compared differences in patients with insomnia to good sleeper controls (i.e., no insomnia history), but not in comparison to fear states (e.g., subjects experiencing acute environmental threats). Put differently, when differences were observed, it was unclear whether the magnitude of the differences observed represented a level of activation that could preclude sleep or whether the observed tonic activation simply represented one factor, of several, responsible for protracted difficulties with sleep initiation and maintenance [70]. This distinction is important as increases above what is normal or average may be statistically significant, but not necessarily clinically meaningful. One approach to clarifying this issue would be to assess the "hyperarousal" of acute and chronic insomnia (across multiple indices) and to compare such data with experimentally elicited startle or fear responses. In this way, the scale of the arousal could be "biocalibrated" and this would allow for inferences about when "hyperarousal" may or may not account for sleeplessness. Alternatively, another approach is to use more naturalistic studies that estimate the level of hyperarousal required to prohibit sleep. For example, findings from two classical studies on ship engineers during on-call periods showed that high-stress/high-anticipation situations can disturb the subjective and objective quality of sleep [71,72].

Three additional important considerations when investigating the association between insomnia and hyperarousal are that (1) daytime indices of hyperarousal may be unrelated to nocturnal indices of hyperarousal (and insomnia may be about one or both), (2) the relative impact of wakefulness at night should be taken into consideration when conceptualizing the effect of hyperarousal, and (3) the association between insomnia and hyperarousal may vary with regard to insomnia type and/or sub-type. With regard to diurnal/nocturnal differences, the neural or hormonal indices that are overactive during sleep (e.g., increases in high frequency EEG activity [51,53]), suggesting a state of hyperarousal) may be separate and distinct from those that are overactive during wakefulness (e.g., increases in glucocorticoids [73–75]). Put differently, evidence that supports hyperarousal during one phase (e.g., daytime) or state (e.g., wake), does not necessitate that hyperarousal also be present during other phases/states. With regard to nocturnal wakefulness, it is unclear whether the group differences in hyperarousal observed during sleep, such as increased EEG activity, metabolic rate, or hormonal secretion [49,50], are related to condition (i.e., insomnia disorder) or whether they are related to other factors. It is possible, for example, that these differences observed at night are better explained by time spent awake, and not any insomnia-related disease process. Future work should, therefore, account for the extent to which hyperarousal varies as a function of nocturnal wakefulness, as compared to insomnia diagnosis. Finally, it may be the case that hyperarousal is more characteristic of certain types (e.g., CI with objective short sleep duration phenotype [76]) or sub-types of insomnia (initial, middle, and late insomnia [66]), and, therefore, these differences should be accounted for in future research.

6. Hyperarousal May Apply to Acute but not Chronic Insomnia

If acute insomnia is genuinely a part of the fight/flight response (i.e., an override to the normal two-process regulation of sleep timing, depth, and/or duration), it follows that hyperarousal is the mechanism by which adaptive sleeplessness is ensured. That is, under unsafe conditions, sleep is naturally inhibited. In the case of CI, while it is logical that the precipitant for sleeplessness may be the same, it is unlikely given that fight/flight levels of hyperarousal may only be sustained for minutes to hours. Thus, the emergent question is whether chronic hyperarousal (e.g., tonic activation of the autonomic nervous system and adrenal cortex) is sufficient to produce sleeplessness by itself or in combination with other factors. The concern, however, is that past research has, in most cases, assumed this to be true. Recent research has been so focused on identifying *the* marker of hyperarousal in insomnia, its reliance on theory and making theory-driven hypotheses has wavered. That is, what markers of hyperarousal, and in what context, are investigators evaluating and are these markers consistent with the theoretical models regarding the etiology and pathophysiology of insomnia? Let's take hypercortisolemia as an example. One possible explanation for the pathophysiology of insomnia is that CI results from excessive CNS activation [53,77–80]. The identified substrates for excessive CNS activation have been related to catecholaminergic function and/or HPA axis dysregulation, in the form of increased cortisol secretion [81]. Theoretically this seems plausible given what was discussed above regarding the acute sleeplessness that naturally occurs in response to a perceived or real threat. The scientific literature on hypercortisolemia as an index for hyperarousal in chronic insomnia is surprisingly mixed [66,73,82–87]. The primary issue here is that the definition of hypercortisolemia has been inconsistent across studies [67]. Like most other biological systems, the HPA axis is dynamic, with multiple regulatory inputs [88,89], and, therefore, no two measures of HPA axis functioning (or the resultant cortisol secretion) are the same. For example, cortisol secretion at night while one is asleep has a very different regulatory function than the subsequent cortisol awakening response (CAR) [90]. Comparisons between these two indices, in the context of insomnia, are, therefore, difficult to interpret. The overarching point is that our measures of hyperarousal must be theoretically derived. It is not enough to implicate a biological system in the pathophysiology of insomnia and then measure its association using established methods, but without consideration to whether those methods are consistent with theory (e.g., there's minimal conceptual rationale for observing group differences in CAR among patients with CI) [74,91].

All this said, a conservative reading of the behavioral models of insomnia suggest that acute hyperarousal is sufficient to precipitate acute insomnia but that chronic hyperarousal is not sufficient to serve as a perpetuating factor for chronic insomnia. The behavioral models (i.e., the 3P and 4P renditions) suggest that chronic insomnia occurs largely in association with behavioral factors (e.g., sleep extension or being awake for extended periods of time in the bed and bedroom) and that with time insomnia occurs as "conditioned" wakefulness. Thus, it may be the case that AI is precipitated by hyperarousal and that CI is perpetuated, to some extent by tonic activation of the fight/flight system, but in larger measure by conditioned wakefulness and/or the failure to inhibit wakefulness [92]. If true, it would be expected that AI would show dramatic elevations on measures of sympathetic activation, while CI would only show modest elevations as compared to what is typical of good sleep.

Conditioned wakefulness is related to poor stimulus control, or the act of engaging in nonsleep-related behaviors in bed (or the bedroom) or being awake while in bed for extended periods of time. These behaviors result in conditioned wakefulness, which refers to the notion that the induction of the physiology of wakefulness, for example, during the anticipation of sleep, is due to an environmental precipitant. An environmentally conditioned stimulus (CS) produces the conditioned response (CR) of insomnia [93,94]. This CR may also occur during sleep, which may explain why individuals with insomnia are quicker to wake up (i.e., the latency to transition out of the physiological state of sleep may be shorter) and experience more prolonged awakenings during the night (i.e., the probability of a brief interruption in sleep to lead to a full-blown awakening is greater). It is possible that there may be a role for hyperarousal here, in that the environmental CS may elicit a conditioned (physiological) stress response (e.g., an acute increase in HPA/adrenergic hormones or pulse) and that this may in turn elicit conditioned wakefulness. It is important, however, to distinguish this from a true fear response, in that this "stress response" is likely not at that level but only incrementally higher than baseline (normal), but enough to elicit wakefulness. Given some perspectives that insomnia is characterized by a hybrid brain state (localized wakefulness during otherwise global sleep) [95,96], it may also be the case that these psychobiological responses are producing localized wakefulness, which may contribute to the high prevalence of sleep-state misperception in patients with insomnia, or the phenomenon that an individual perceives oneself to be awake (retrospectively), despite being classified (polysomnographically) as being asleep. This said, rather than "hyperarousal", CI may be better characterized by disinhibition of wakefulness or a failure to inhibit wakefulness during times of sleep or a disconnect between systems that are supposed to be online/offline during wake/sleep (i.e., maladaptive conditioning) [92,95].

7. Where to from Here?

The goal of the present theoretical review is three-fold: (1) To provide a clear definition for acute and chronic insomnia, based on the available nosological manuals and the scientific literature, with a special emphasis on the limitations of these definitions; (2) to provide a clear definition for hyperarousal, as it relates to insomnia; and (3) to proffer the perspective that the two beliefs described at the opening of this paper are not necessarily true, or at least, that the relationship between acute and chronic insomnia (and hyperarousal) is more complex than previously believed. This alternative perspective suggests that AI and CI are not necessarily different points in the natural history of insomnia (disorder), but rather that they are distinct states. More, there is no clear evidence to support that the severity and frequency of AI and CI are the same (it may be the case that AI is a brief yet more intense version of CI) and/or that the biopsychosocial concomitants of AI and CI are the same. While the symptom profiles for the two are the same (at least from a theoretical perspective), the etiology and pathophysiology of each are likely very different, and specifically AI may be more about "hyperarousal", whereas CI may be more related to other processes, such as homeostatic dysregulation and/or conditioned wakefulness. It is possible that these processes are related to traditional indices of hyperarousal. However, we argue here that the use of the term "hyperarousal" may be a misrepresentation of the magnitude of these responses and that the hyperarousal observed in CI may be different than the hyperarousal observed in AI, and importantly, that these two should not be conflated.

Based on the current state of the science, the following recommendations are offered, with the intention that they could potentially guide future research efforts:

(1) Natural history of insomnia data should be used to define what constitutes the temporal stages of insomnia. Note: It seems likely that such data will need to capture normal variation in sleep continuity, acute sleeplessness, persistent poor sleep, and chronic insomnia (e.g., Insomnia Disorder).

(2) The temporal stages of insomnia should be compared regarding incident frequency and severity (i.e., does sleep continuity disturbance occur on more days per week and/or with greater average severity when the insomnia is normative vs. acute vs. persistent vs. chronic?).

(3) Multi-method, multi-trait type studies of insomnia should be used to define when "acute hyperarousal" (fight-or-fight responding) is and is not solely responsible for the occurrence of difficulties initiating and maintaining sleep.

(4) Experimental assays or protocols should be developed to distinguish between sleeplessness due to hyperarousal and insomnia due to conditioned wakefulness and/or the failure to inhibit wakefulness.

Author Contributions: Conceptualization, I.V., J.G.E., and M.L.P.; writing—original draft preparation, I.V., A.M.N., A.M., and M.L.P.; writing—review and editing, I.V., A.M.N., A.M., C.H.B., J.G.E., and M.L.P. All authors have read and agreed to the published version of the manuscript.

Funding: This research received no external funding.

Acknowledgments: Ivan Vargas is currently funded by a National Institutes of Health (NIH) Mentored Patient-Oriented Research Career Development Award (K23HL141581). Michael L. Perlis is currently funded by an NIH Midcareer Investigator Award (K24AG055602).

Conflicts of Interest: The authors declare no conflict of interest.

References

1. Centers A of SD, Sleep A for the PS of Sleep Disorders Classification Committee, Association of Sleep Disorders Centers. Sleep. Available online: https://academic.oup.com/sleep/article-lookup/doi/10.1093/sleep/2.1.1 (accessed on 17 December 2019).

2. DSM-5 American Psychiatric Association. *Diagnostic and Statistical Manual of Mental Disorders*; American Psychiatric Association: Washington, DC, USA, 1980.

3. American Academy of Sleep Medicine. The International Classification of Sleep Disorders: Diagnostic and Coding Manual. In *The International Classification of Sleep Disorders: Diagnostic and Coding Manual*, 2nd ed.; American Academy of Sleep Medicine: Chicago, IL, USA, 2001.

4. NIH State of the Science Conference Statement on Manifestations and Management of Chronic Insomnia in Adults Statement. *J. Clin. Sleep Med.* **2005**, *1*, 412–421. [CrossRef]

5. Roth, T.; Roehrs, T. Insomnia: epidemiology, characteristics, and consequences. *Clin. Cornerstone* **2003**, *5*, 5–15. [CrossRef]

6. Ellis, J.G.; Gehrman, P.; Espie, C.A.; Riemann, D.; Perlis, M.L. Acute insomnia: Current conceptualizations and future directions. *Sleep Med. Rev.* **2012**, *16*, 5–14. [CrossRef] [PubMed]

7. Spielman, A.J.; Glovinsky, P.B. The varied nature of insomnia. In *Case Studies in Insomnia*; Springer: Boston, MA, USA, 1991; pp. 1–18.

8. Spielman, A.J.; Glovinsky, P.B. The diagnostic interview and differential diagnosis for complaints of insomnia. In *Understanding Sleep: The Evaluation and Treatment of Sleep Disorders*; American Psychological Association (APA): Washington, DC, USA, 1997; pp. 125–160.

9. Morin, C.M.; Bélanger, L.; LeBlanc, M.; Ivers, H.; Savard, J.; Espie, C.A.; Merette, C.; Baillargeon, L.; Gregoire, J.P. The natural history of insomnia a population-based 3-year longitudinal study. *Arch. Intern. Med.* **2009**, *169*, 447–453. [CrossRef] [PubMed]

10. Leblanc, M.; Mérette, C.; Savard, J.; Ivers, H.; Baillargeon, L.; Morin, C.M. Incidence and Risk Factors of Insomnia in a Population-Based Sample. *Sleep* **2009**, *32*, 1027–1037. [CrossRef] [PubMed]

11. DSM-5 American Psychiatric Association. *Diagnostic and Statistical Manual of Mental Disorders: DSM-IV-TR*; American Psychiatric Association: Washington, DC, USA, 2000.

12. American Psychiatric Association. *Diagnostic and Statistical Manual of Mental Disorders (DSM-5®)*; American Psychiatric Pub: Arlington, TX, USA, 2013; p. 866.

13. Ellis, J.G.; Perlis, M.L.; Neale, L.F.; Espie, C.A.; Bastien, C.H. The natural history of insomnia: Focus on prevalence and incidence of acute insomnia. *J. Psychiatr. Res.* **2012**, *46*, 1278–1285. [CrossRef]

14. Perlis, M.L.; Vargas, I.; Ellis, J.G.; A Grandner, M.; Morales, K.H.; Gencarelli, A.; Khader, W.; Kloss, J.D.; Gooneratne, N.S.; E Thase, M. The Natural History of Insomnia: the incidence of acute insomnia and subsequent progression to chronic insomnia or recovery in good sleeper subjects. *Sleep* **2019**. [CrossRef]

15. Harvey, A.G. Insomnia: Symptom or diagnosis? *Clin. Psychol. Rev.* **2001**, *21*, 1037–1059. [CrossRef]

16. Taylor, D.J.; Lichstein, K.L.; Durrence, H.H.; Reidel, B.W.; Bush, A.J. Epidemiology of insomnia, depression, and anxiety. *Sleep* **2005**, *28*, 1457–1464. [CrossRef]

17. A Borbély, A. A two process model of sleep regulation. *Hum. Neurobiol.* **1982**, *1*, 195–204.

18. Perlis, M.; Shaw, P.J.; Cano, G.; Espie, C.A. Models of Insomnia. In *Principles and Practice of Sleep Medicine*; Elsevier BV: Amsterdam, The Netherlands, 2011; pp. 850–865.

19. Morin, C.M.; Benca, R. Chronic insomnia. *Lancet* **2012**, *379*, 1129–1141. [CrossRef]

20. American Academy of Sleep Medicine. *International Classification of Sleep Disorders—Third Edition (ICSD-3)*; American Academy of Sleep Medicine: Darien, IL, USA, 2014.

21. International Classification of Diseases (ICD). Available online: http://www.who.int/classifications/icd/en/ (accessed on 11 May 2012).

22. Pigeon, W.R.; Hegel, M.; Unützer, J.; Fan, M.-Y.; Sateia, M.J.; Lyness, J.M.; Phillips, C.; Perlis, M.L. Is Insomnia a Perpetuating Factor for Late-Life Depression in the IMPACT Cohort? *Sleep* **2008**, *31*, 481–488. [CrossRef] [PubMed]

23. Buckley, T.M.; Schatzberg, A.F. On the Interactions of the Hypothalamic-Pituitary-Adrenal (HPA) Axis and Sleep: Normal HPA Axis Activity and Circadian Rhythm, Exemplary Sleep Disorders. *J. Clin. Endocrinol. Metab.* **2005**, *90*, 3106–3114. [CrossRef] [PubMed]

24. Johnson, P.L.; Molosh, A.; Fitz, S.D.; Truitt, W.A.; Shekhar, A. Orexin, stress, and anxiety/panic states. In *Progress in Brain Research*; Elsevier BV: Amsterdam, The Netherlands, 2012; Volume 198, pp. 133–161.

25. Winkelman, J.W.; Buxton, O.M.; Jensen, J.E.; Benson, K.L.; O'Connor, S.P.; Wang, W.; Renshaw, P.F. Reduced Brain GABA in Primary Insomnia: Preliminary Data from 4T Proton Magnetic Resonance Spectroscopy (1H-MRS). *Sleep* **2008**, *31*, 1499–1506. [CrossRef] [PubMed]

26. Ford, D.E. Epidemiologic study of sleep disturbances and psychiatric disorders. An opportunity for prevention? *JAMA* **1989**, *262*, 1479–1484. [CrossRef]

27. Ohayon, M.M. Epidemiology of insomnia: what we know and what we still need to learn. *Sleep Med. Rev.* **2002**, *6*, 97–111. [CrossRef]

28. Morin, C.; Leblanc, M.; Daley, M.; Gregoire, J.-P.; Merette, C. Epidemiology of insomnia: Prevalence, self-help treatments, consultations, and determinants of help-seeking behaviors. *Sleep Med.* **2006**, *7*, 123–130. [CrossRef]

29. Chung, K.-F.; Yeung, W.-F.; Ho, F.Y.-Y.; Yung, K.-P.; Yu, Y.-M.; Kwok, C.-W. Cross-cultural and comparative epidemiology of insomnia: The Diagnostic and Statistical Manual (DSM), International Classification of Diseases (ICD) and International Classification of Sleep Disorders (ICSD). *Sleep Med.* **2015**, *16*, 477–482. [CrossRef] [PubMed]

30. Foley, D.J.; Monjan, A.; Simonsick, E.M.; Wallace, R.B.; Blazer, D.G. Incidence and remission of insomnia among elderly adults: an epidemiologic study of 6,800 persons over three years. *Sleep* **1999**, *22*.

31. Gureje, O.; Oladeji, B.D.; Abiona, T.; Makanjuola, V.; Esan, O. The Natural History of Insomnia in the Ibadan Study of Ageing. *Sleep* **2011**, *34*, 965–973. [CrossRef]

32. Romero, L.M.; Butler, L.K. Endocrinology of stress. *Int. J. Comp. Psychol.* **2007**, *20*, 89–95.

33. Papadimitriou, A.; Priftis, K.N. Regulation of the hypothalamic-pituitary-adrenal axis. Available online: https://www.researchgate.net/publication/26335151 (accessed on 17 December 2019).

34. Bracha, H.S. Freeze, Flight, Fight, Fright, Faint: Adaptationist Perspectives on the Acute Stress Response Spectrum. *CNS Spectrums* **2004**, *9*, 679–685. [CrossRef] [PubMed]

35. Chrousos, G.P. The concepts of stress and stress system disorders. Overview of physical and behavioral homeostasis. *JAMA* **1992**, *267*, 1244–1252. [CrossRef]

36. Tsigos, C.; Chrousos, G.P. Hypothalamic–pituitary–adrenal axis, neuroendocrine factors and stress. *J. Psychosom. Res.* **2002**, *53*, 865–871. [CrossRef]

37. Myers, B.; McKlveen, J.M.; Herman, J.P. Neural regulation of the stress response: The many faces of feedback. Available online: http://www.scielo.br/scielo.php?pid=S0100-879X2012000400002&script=sci_arttext&tlng=es (accessed on 17 December 2019).

38. Jones, M.T.; Tiptaft, E.M.; Brush, F.R.; Fergusson, D.A.N.; Neame, R.L.B. Evidence for dual corticosteroid-receptor mechanisms in the feedback control of adrenocorticotrophin secretion. *J. Endocrinol.* **1974**, *60*, 223–233. [CrossRef] [PubMed]

39. Jacobs, N.; Myin-Germeys, I.; Derom, C.; Delespaul, P.; Van Os, J.; Nicolson, N. A momentary assessment study of the relationship between affective and adrenocortical stress responses in daily life. *Boil. Psychol.* **2007**, *74*, 60–66. [CrossRef]

40. McHale, S.M.; Blocklin, M.K.; Walter, K.N.; Davis, K.D.; Almeida, D.M.; Klein, L.C. The role of daily activities in youths' stress physiology. *J. Adolesc. Heal.* **2012**, *51*, 623–628. [CrossRef]

41. Smyth, J.; Ockenfels, M.C.; Porter, L.; Kirschbaum, C.; Hellhammer, D.H.; A Stone, A. Stressors and mood measured on a momentary basis are associated with salivary cortisol secretion. *Psychoneuroendocrinology* **1998**, *23*, 353–370. [CrossRef]

42. Wassing, R.; Benjamins, J.S.; Dekker, K.; Moens, S.; Spiegelhalder, K.; Feige, B.; Riemann, D.; Van Der Sluis, S.; Van Der Werf, Y.D.; Talamini, L.M.; et al. Slow dissolving of emotional distress contributes to hyperarousal. *Proc. Natl. Acad. Sci. USA* **2016**, *113*, 2538–2543. [CrossRef]

43. Wassing, R.; Benjamins, J.S.; Talamini, L.M.; Schalkwijk, F.; Van Someren, E.J.W. Overnight worsening of emotional distress indicates maladaptive sleep in insomnia. *Sleep* **2019**, *42*, 1–8. [CrossRef]

44. Osuch, E.A.; Willis, M.W.; Bluhm, R.; Ursano, R.J.; Drevets, W.C. CSTS Neuroimaging Study Group Neurophysiological responses to traumatic reminders in the acute aftermath of serious motor vehicle collisions using [15O]-H2O positron emission tomography. *Boil. Psychiatry* **2008**, *64*, 327–335. [CrossRef]

45. Germain, A.; Buysse, D.J.; Nofzinger, E. Sleep-specific mechanisms underlying posttraumatic stress disorder: Integrative review and neurobiological hypotheses. *Sleep Med. Rev.* **2008**, *12*, 185–195. [CrossRef]

46. Dhabhar, F.S.; McEwen, B.S.; Spencer, R.L. Adaptation to prolonged or repeated stress–comparison between rat strains showing intrinsic differences in reactivity to acute stress. *Neuroendocrinology* **1997**, *65*, 360–368. [CrossRef]

47. Ockenfels, M.C.; Porter, L.; Smyth, J.; Kirschbaum, C.; Hellhammer, D.H.; A Stone, A. Effect of chronic stress associated with unemployment on salivary cortisol: overall cortisol levels, diurnal rhythm, and acute stress reactivity. *Psychosom. Med.* **1995**, *57*, 460–467. [CrossRef]

48. Shields, G.S.; Sazma, M.A.; McCullough, A.M.; Yonelinas, A.P. The effects of acute stress on episodic memory: A meta-analysis and integrative review. *Psychol. Bull.* **2017**, *143*, 636–675. [CrossRef]

49. Riemann, D.; Spiegelhalder, K.; Feige, B.; Voderholzer, U.; Berger, M.; Perlis, M.; Nissen, C. The hyperarousal model of insomnia: A review of the concept and its evidence. *Sleep Med. Rev.* **2010**, *14*, 19–31. [CrossRef] [PubMed]

50. Spiegelhalder, K.; Riemann, D. Hyperarousal and insomnia. *Sleep Med. Clin.* **2013**, *12*, 299–307. [CrossRef]

51. Perlis, M.L.; Merica, H.; Smith, M.T.; Giles, N.E. Beta EEG activity and insomnia. *Sleep Med. Rev.* **2001**, *5*, 365–376. [CrossRef] [PubMed]

52. Perlis, M.L.; Smith, M.T.; Orff, H.J.; Andrews, P.J.; E Giles, D. The mesograde amnesia of sleep may be attenuated in subjects with primary insomnia. *Physiol. Behav.* **2001**, *74*, 71–76. [CrossRef]

53. Perlis, M.L.; Smith, M.T.; Andrews, P.J.; Orff, H.J.; Giles, D.E. Beta / Gamma EEG Activity in Patients with Primary and and Secondary Insomnia and Good Sleeper Controls. *Sleep* **2001**, *24*, 110–117. [CrossRef]

54. Spiegelhalder, K.; Regen, W.; Feige, B.; Holz, J.; Piosczyk, H.; Baglioni, C.; Riemann, D.; Nissen, C. Increased EEG sigma and beta power during NREM sleep in primary insomnia. *Boil. Psychol.* **2012**, *91*, 329–333. [CrossRef]

55. Devoto, A.; Violani, C.; Lucidi, F.; Lombardo, C. P300 amplitude in subjects with primary insomnia is modulated by their sleep quality. *J. Psychosom. Res.* **2003**, *54*, 3–10. [CrossRef]

56. Devoto, A.; Manganelli, S.; Lucidi, F.; Lombardo, C.; Russo, P.M.; Violani, C. Quality of sleep and P300 amplitude in primary insomnia: a preliminary study. *Sleep* **2005**, *28*, 859–863. [CrossRef] [PubMed]

57. Nofzinger, E.A.; Buysse, D.J.; Germain, A.; Price, J.C.; Miewald, J.M.; Kupfer, D.J. Functional Neuroimaging Evidence for Hyperarousal in Insomnia. *Am. J. Psychiatry* **2004**, *161*, 2126–2128. [CrossRef] [PubMed]

58. Plante, D.T.; Jensen, J.E.; Schoerning, L.; Winkelman, J.W. Reduced γ-Aminobutyric Acid in Occipital and Anterior Cingulate Cortices in Primary Insomnia: A Link to Major Depressive Disorder? *Neuropsychopharmacology* **2012**, *37*, 1548–1557. [CrossRef] [PubMed]

59. Plante, D.T.; Jensen, J.E.; Winkelman, J.W. The role of GABA in primary insomnia. *Sleep* **2012**, *35*, 741–742. [CrossRef]

60. Stepanski, E.; Glinn, M.; Zorick, F.; Roehrs, T.; Roth, T. Heart rate changes in chronic insomnia. *Stress Med.* **1994**, *10*, 261–266. [CrossRef]

61. Bonnet, M.H.; Arand, D.L. Heart rate variability in insomniacs and matched normal sleepers. *Psychosom. Med.* **1998**, *60*, 610–615. [CrossRef]

62. Broman, J.-E.; Hetta, J. Electrodermal activity in patients with persistent insomnia. *J. Sleep Res.* **1994**, *3*, 165–170. [CrossRef]

63. Irwin, M.; Clark, C.; Kennedy, B.; Gillin, J.C.; Ziegler, M. Nocturnal catecholamines and immune function in insomniacs, depressed patients, and control subjects. *Brain Behav. Immun.* **2003**, *17*, 365–372. [CrossRef]

64. Lack, L.C.; Gradisar, M.; Van Someren, E.J.W.; Wright, H.R.; Lushington, K. The relationship between insomnia and body temperatures. *Sleep Med. Rev.* **2008**, *12*, 307–317. [CrossRef] [PubMed]

65. Bonnet, M.H.; Arand, D.L. 24-Hour Metabolic Rate in Insomniacs and Matched Normal Sleepers. *Sleep* **1995**, *18*, 581–588. [CrossRef] [PubMed]

66. Vgontzas, A.N.; Bixler, E.O.; Lin, H.M.; Prolo, P.; Mastorakos, G.; Vela-Bueno, A.; Kales, A.; Chrousos, G.P. Chronic Insomnia Is Associated with Nyctohemeral Activation of the Hypothalamic-Pituitary-Adrenal Axis: Clinical Implications. *J. Clin. Endocrinol. Metab.* **2001**, *86*, 3787–3794. [CrossRef]

67. Vargas, I.; Vgontzas, A.N.; Abelson, J.L.; Faghih, R.T.; Morales, K.H.; Perlis, M.L. Altered ultradian cortisol rhythmicity as a potential neurobiologic substrate for chronic insomnia. *Sleep Med. Rev.* **2018**, *41*, 234–243. [CrossRef]

68. Stepanski, E.; Zorick, F.; Roehrs, T.; Young, D.; Roth, T.; Edward, S.; Frank, Z.; Timothy, R.; David, Y.; Thomas, R. Daytime Alertness in Patients with Chronic Insomnia Compared with Asymptomatic Control Subjects. *Sleep* **1988**, *11*, 54–60. [CrossRef]

69. Roehrs, T.A.; Randall, S.; Harris, E.; Maan, R.; Roth, T. MSLT in Primary Insomnia: Stability and Relation to Nocturnal Sleep. *Sleep* **2011**, *34*, 1647–1652. [CrossRef]

70. Bonnet, M.H. Hyperarousal as the basis for insomnia: Effect size and significance. *Sleep* **2005**, *24*, 1500–1501. [CrossRef]

71. Torsvall, L.; Åkerstedt, T. Disturbed Sleep While Being On-Call: An EEG Study of Ships' Engineers. *Sleep* **1988**, *11*, 35–38. [CrossRef]

72. Torsvall, L.; Castenfors, K.; Åkerstedt, T.; Fröberg, J. Sleep at sea: a diary study of the effects of unattended machinery space watch duty. *Ergonomycs* **1987**, *30*, 1335–1340. [CrossRef]

73. Xia, L.; Chen, G.-H.; Li, Z.-H.; Jiang, S.; Shen, J. Alterations in Hypothalamus-Pituitary-Adrenal/Thyroid Axes and Gonadotropin-Releasing Hormone in the Patients with Primary Insomnia: A Clinical Research. *PLOS ONE* **2013**, *8*, e71065. [CrossRef]

74. Zhang, J.; Lam, S.-P.; Li, S.X.; Ma, R.C.W.; Kong, A.P.S.; Chan, M.H.M.; Ho, C.-S.; Li, A.M.; Wing, Y.-K. A Community-Based Study on the Association Between Insomnia and Hypothalamic-Pituitary-Adrenal Axis: Sex and Pubertal Influences. *J. Clin. Endocrinol. Metab.* **2014**, *99*, 2277–2287. [CrossRef] [PubMed]

75. Floam, S.; Simpson, N.; Nemeth, E.; Scott-Sutherland, J.; Gautam, S.; Haack, M. Sleep characteristics as predictor variables of stress systems markers in insomnia disorder. *J. Sleep Res.* **2015**, *24*, 296–304. [CrossRef] [PubMed]

76. Vgontzas, A.N.; Fernandez-Mendoza, J.; Liao, D.; Bixler, E.O. Insomnia with objective short sleep duration: the most biologically severe phenotype of the disorder. *Sleep Med. Rev.* **2013**, *17*, 241–254. [CrossRef] [PubMed]

77. Nofzinger, E.A.; Buysse, D.J.; Germain, A.; Price, J.; Miewald, J.; Kupfer, D.J. Insomnia: Functional neuroimaging evidence for hyperarousal. *Sleep* **2004**, *27*, 272. [CrossRef] [PubMed]

78. Merica, H.; Blois, R.; Gaillard, J.-M. Spectral characteristics of sleep EEG in chronic insomnia. *Eur. J. Neurosci.* **1998**, *10*, 1826–1834. [CrossRef]

79. Merica, H.; Gaillard, J.-M. The EEG of the sleep onset period in insomnia: A discriminant analysis. *Physiol. Behav.* **1992**, *52*, 199–204. [CrossRef]

80. Lamarche, C.H.; Ogilvie, R.D. Electrophysiological changes during the sleep onset period of psychophysiological insomniacs, psychiatric insomniacs, and normal sleepers. *Sleep* **1997**, *20*, 726–733. [CrossRef]

81. Perlis, M.; Gehrman, P.; Pigeon, W.R.; Findley, J.; Drummond, S.; Pigeon, W.; Gehrman, P.; Findley, J. Neurobiological Mechanisms In Chronic Insomnia. *Sleep Med. Clin.* **2009**, *4*, 549–558. [CrossRef] [PubMed]

82. Backhaus, J.; Junghanns, K.; Hohagen, F. Sleep disturbances are correlated with decreased morning awakening salivary cortisol. *Psychoneuroendocrinology* **2004**, *29*, 1184–1191. [CrossRef]

83. Backhaus, J.; Junghanns, K.; Born, J.; Hohaus, K.; Faasch, F.; Hohagen, F. Impaired Declarative Memory Consolidation During Sleep in Patients With Primary Insomnia: Influence of Sleep Architecture and Nocturnal Cortisol Release. *Boil. Psychiatry* **2006**, *60*, 1324–1330. [CrossRef]

84. Vgontzas, A.N.; Tsigos, C.; O Bixler, E.; A Stratakis, C.; Zachman, K.; Kales, A.; Vela-Bueno, A.; Chrousos, G.P. Chronic insomnia and activity of the stress system: a preliminary study. *J. Psychosom. Res.* **1998**, *45*, 21–31. [CrossRef]

85. Riemann, D.; Klein, T.; Rodenbeck, A.; Feige, B.; Horny, A.; Hummel, R.; Weske, G.; Al-Shajlawi, A.; Voderholzer, U. Nocturnal cortisol and melatonin secretion in primary insomnia. *Psychiatry Res. Neuroimaging* **2002**, *113*, 17–27. [CrossRef]

86. Rodenbeck, A.; Huether, G.; Rüther, E.; Hajak, G. Interactions between evening and nocturnal cortisol secretion and sleep parameters in patients with severe chronic primary insomnia. *Neurosci. Lett.* **2002**, *324*, 159–163. [CrossRef]

87. Varkevisser, M.; Van Dongen, H.P.; Kerkhof, G.A. Physiologic indexes in chronic insomnia during a constant routine: evidence for general hyperarousal? *Sleep* **2005**, *28*, 1588–1596. [PubMed]

88. Cook, N. The physiology of sleep: Homeostasis and health. *Br. J. Wellbeing* **2010**, *1*, 16–20. [CrossRef]

89. Datta, S.; MacLean, R.R. Neurobiological mechanisms for the regulation of mammalian sleep-wake behavior: Reinterpretation of historical evidence and inclusion of contemporary cellular and molecular evidence. *Neur. Biobehav. Rev.* **2007**, *31*, 775–824. [CrossRef]

90. Elder, G.J.; Wetherell, M.A.; Barclay, N.L.; Ellis, J.G. The cortisol awakening response–applications and implications for sleep medicine. *Sleep Med. Rev.* **2013**, *18*, 215–224. [CrossRef]

91. Zhang, J.; Ma, R.C.; Kong, A.P.; So, W.Y.; Li, A.M.; Lam, S.P.; Li, S.X.; Yu, M.W.; Ho, C.S.; Chan, M.H.; et al. Relationship of Sleep Quantity and Quality with 24-Hour Urinary Catecholamines and Salivary Awakening Cortisol in Healthy Middle-Aged Adults. *Sleep* **2011**, *34*, 225–233. [CrossRef]

92. Espie, C.A. Insomnia: Conceptual Issues in the Development, Persistence, and Treatment of Sleep Disorder in Adults. *Annu. Rev. Psychol.* **2002**, *53*, 215–243. [CrossRef]

93. Bootzin, R.R. Stimulus Control Treatment for Insomnia. *Am. Psychol. Assoc. A. Hist. Perspect.* **1972**, *7*, 395–396.

94. Perlis, M.L.; E Giles, D.; Mendelson, W.B.; Bootzin, R.R.; Wyatt, J.K. Psychophysiological insomnia: the behavioural model and a neurocognitive perspective. *J. Sleep Res.* **1997**, *6*, 179–188. [CrossRef] [PubMed]
95. Buysse, D.J.; Germain, A.; Hall, M.; Monk, T.H.; Nofzinger, E.A. A Neurobiological Model of Insomnia. *Drug Discov. Today: Dis. Model.* **2011**, *8*, 129–137. [CrossRef] [PubMed]
96. Tononi, G.; Cirelli, C. Sleep and the Price of Plasticity: From Synaptic and Cellular Homeostasis to Memory Consolidation and Integration. *Neuron. Cell Press* **2014**, *81*, 12–34. [CrossRef] [PubMed]

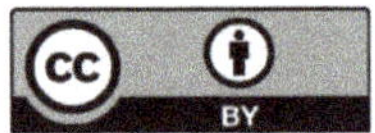

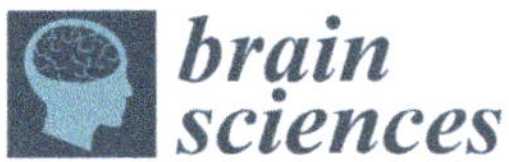 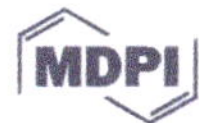

Article

Hyperarousal Is Associated with Socioemotional Processing in Individuals with Insomnia Symptoms and Good Sleepers

Reuben D. M. Howlett, Kari A. Lustig, Kevin J. MacDonald and Kimberly A. Cote *

Psychology Department, Brock University, 1812 Sir Isaac Brock Way, St. Catharines, ON L2S 3A1, Canada;
rh16yq@brocku.ca (R.D.M.H.); kl14qc@brocku.ca (K.A.L.); km11pv@brocku.ca (K.J.M.)
* Correspondence: kcote@brocku.ca; Tel.: +1-905-688-5550 (ext. 4806); Fax: +1-905-688-6922

Received: 14 January 2020; Accepted: 18 February 2020; Published: 20 February 2020

Abstract: Despite complaints of difficulties in waking socioemotional functioning by individuals with insomnia, only a few studies have investigated emotion processing performance in this group. Additionally, the role of sleep in socioemotional processing has not been investigated extensively nor using quantitative measures of sleep. Individuals with insomnia symptoms ($n = 14$) and healthy good sleepers ($n = 15$) completed two nights of at-home polysomnography, followed by an afternoon of in-lab performance testing on tasks measuring the processing of emotional facial expressions. The insomnia group self-reported less total sleep time, but no other group differences in sleep or task performance were observed. Greater beta EEG power throughout the night was associated with higher intensity ratings of happy, fearful and sad faces for individuals with insomnia, yet blunted sensitivity and lower accuracy for good sleepers. Thus, the presence of hyperarousal differentially impacted socioemotional processing of faces in individuals with insomnia symptoms and good sleepers.

Keywords: insomnia; hyperarousal; emotion processing

---

1. Introduction

The capacity to function well in daytime life is dependent on a night of quality sleep. Approximately 10%–15% of the population suffers from chronic poor sleep due to insomnia, a chronic condition characterized by difficulty initiating and/or maintaining sleep [1–4]. Insomnia leads to daytime performance deficits in cognitive abilities such as memory, attention, and concentration, and several of these performance deficits have been linked to poor sleep [5–11]. Another feature of insomnia is reports of reduced social engagement [12–14], suggesting that one consequence of insomnia is poor social functioning. However, little research has examined the processing of socioemotional content in patients with insomnia, despite complaints of daytime impairment in these areas (e.g., [12,15]), and the literature showing that both experimental sleep deprivation and insomnia lead to alterations and/or impairments in emotion processing (for reviews, see [16,17]).

There is some evidence to suggest a role for sleep in waking emotion processing in insomnia. Less time in SWS and REM sleep has been linked to heightened amygdala reactivity to intense negative emotion stimuli [18]. Moreover, the functional connectivity of orbitofrontal areas (a region of emotion processing) was also positively associated with complaints of poorer sleep history [19]. Waking differences in the activity of the fusiform gyrus, a region associated with the processing of faces, have also been linked to subjective reports of historic poor sleep quality and greater symptom duration of insomnia [20]. Findings of altered relative glucose metabolism, in sleep relative to wake, in regions associated with salience and emotion processing in individuals with insomnia [21,22], suggest that the cortical activation of these regions may continue to be engaged and/or uninhibited during sleep, potentially taxing cognitive resources for next-day emotion processing and functioning.

Following from this imaging work, the severity of sleep impairment experienced by individuals with insomnia may be associated with the extent of waking impairment in emotion processing.

Only a few studies have investigated waking emotion processing in individuals with insomnia. Baglioni and colleagues reported that insomnia patients showed greater physiological response to emotional picture scenes using measures of facial EMG and heart rate [23]. Subjectively they rated negative sleep-related stimuli as more unpleasant and arousing. In a subsequent fMRI study, insomnia patients showed a heightened amygdala response to insomnia-related negative picture stimuli, which was interpreted as evidence for a negativity bias towards stimuli of salience [18]. Two recent studies more directly addressed waking socioemotional processing in insomnia by measuring categorization accuracy and intensity judgements when viewing emotionally expressive faces [24,25]. Cronlein and colleagues reported that both patients with insomnia and patients with sleep apnea were less accurate than good sleepers at identifying happy and sad faces. Kyle et al. reported that insomnia patients gave lower intensity ratings than good sleeper controls for faces of fear and sadness. Therefore, complaints of poorer social functioning [12,15] might stem from a reduced capacity of individuals with insomnia to correctly identify or be sensitive to the valence of emotional face expressions, which are important cues for socioemotional functioning [24–28]. Neither study by Kyle et al. or Cronlein et al. found support for a role of sleep in waking performance; however, they only reported basic measures of sleep/wake architecture (such as total sleep time and sleep onset latency) related to performance and did not assess more direct measures of EEG power spectra during sleep/wake periods, which may provide additional insight into relationships between sleep physiology and waking performance.

The contributions of sleep to socioemotional processing in individuals with insomnia have not been examined beyond sleep architecture or self-report measures. The limitations of using PSG for quantifying sleep in insomnia have been well documented [29,30]; quantitative EEG measures of sleep offer more sensitive measures of possible alterations in neurophysiological activity in insomnia sleep [31–42]. Several studies have reported greater power in the high-frequency beta (16–35 Hz) and gamma EEG bands (40–70 Hz), which are normally predominant in waking brain wave activity [43] during both sleep onset and non-REM sleep in individuals with insomnia compared to good sleepers [32,35–38,40–42]. Elevated high-frequency EEG activity in patients with insomnia is thought to represent abnormal arousal and enhanced information processing during sleep and a misperception about sleep states. As such, the presence of high-frequency EEG in sleep in patients with insomnia has been described as hyperarousal, underlying the etiology and pathophysiology of the sleep disorder (see [5,39,44–46] for comprehensive reviews on the topic). Quantitative EEG measurement of sleep allows for the investigation of markers of disturbed sleep beyond differences in gross sleep architecture or subjective perceptions of sleep quality.

The central aim of this study was to examine the relationship between sleep physiology and waking emotion processing in patients with insomnia symptoms compared to good sleepers. To do this, we employed one task that measured the ability to accurately categorize emotionally expressive faces and intensity ratings of those faces using a task previously employed in insomnia patients by Kyle et al. [24], and another emotional face processing task that included an additional element of attentional control to increase the cognitive complexity of the task, particularly given that attentional control has been found to be impaired in insomnia [9,47]. Based on previous findings of differences in salience assessment and perceptual accuracy of emotion expressions [24,25] as well as deficits in attention and inhibitory control in insomnia [5,9], we predicted that individuals reporting insomnia symptoms would have poorer accuracy and lower intensity ratings for emotional face expressions, as well as poorer inhibitory control for emotion distractors. We measured sleep quantitatively using an EEG power spectral analysis and an innovative measure of sleep-depth called the Odds-Ratio-Product (ORP; [48]) in order to more precisely assess the role of sleep physiology in emotion processing. Greater levels of high-frequency EEG activity throughout sleep (e.g., [36,39,41]) and findings of altered relative glucose metabolism in sleep/wake states in regions associated with emotion processing in individuals with insomnia [21,22] suggest that regions of emotion processing may have uninhibited/maintained wake-like activity throughout sleep which could lead to a lack of restoration and/or alteration in waking socioemotional processing the following day. Therefore, we expected that measures of disrupted sleep and hyperarousal over the night would be associated with performance differences on emotion processing tasks for individuals with insomnia symptoms.

2. Method

2.1. Participants

Participants with insomnia (INS) met the DSM-5 criteria for diagnosis [49] as well as having an Insomnia Severity Index (ISI; [50]) score greater than seven (i.e., subclinical or greater levels of insomnia symptomology). Eligible INS individuals reported less than 6.5 h of sleep per night on average, greater than 30 min to fall asleep and/or stay awake throughout the night or early morning awakenings without being able to return to sleep, sleep disturbances for at least three nights a week and lasting three or more months, and that their sleep had negative consequences on daily functioning and/or quality of life. These individuals are described herein as having insomnia symptoms because they met the DSM-5 criteria for insomnia, but PSG recording was not carried out to exclude sleep apnea, restless leg syndrome or periodic limb movement disorders (although they did not endorse symptomology on questionnaires). All the participants reported having no other sleep disorders (e.g., sleep apnea, restless leg syndrome), having no psychiatric illnesses (e.g., schizophrenia, depression, anxiety), no history of concussion or head injury, and taking no medication that affects cognition or sleep. They also reported no recent history of trans-meridian travel, shift-work, or smoking.

Of the 45 participants that passed the preliminary screening and completed the in-lab orientation session, two participants were withdrawn due to technical difficulties with the sleep equipment during the nights of home recording (i.e., no PSG data recorded), one good sleeper was omitted from final analysis for failure to comply with instructions to wake up by 8:00 a.m. on the performance testing day and two participants from the INS group were excluded due to inability to remain awake during performance assessment (i.e., no performance data). One good sleeper was removed who scored greater than seven on the ISI, one good sleeper was removed due to an atypical poor night of sleep, and nine good sleepers were removed because they did not comply with the study instructions and severely restricted their time in bed. Fourteen individuals with insomnia symptoms (INS) (10 women, *M* age = 27 years, *SD* = 9.81) and fifteen good sleeper (GS) controls (13 women, *M* age = 25.60 years, *SD* = 9.56) were included in the data analysis. Participants were paid an $60 honorarium for study completion; the INS group received a copy of a home treatment module [51].

2.2. Materials

Face emotion categorization and intensity task (FCI). This task was adapted from the study by Kyle et al. [24]. A variable inter-stimulus fixation point was displayed for 500–800 ms before a face expressing one of four emotions (happy, sad, fearful, angry) was presented for 400 ms. An empty black screen followed each face stimuli and continued until participant response. Participants responded by a keystroke (keyboard number row 1–4) corresponding with each emotion to categorize the face. Participants were then presented, until response, with a 5-point Likert scale to rate the intensity of the face (1 = "Not very intense" to 5 = "Extremely intense") without the face stimuli present. There was a total of 60 trials of each emotion (240 total trials) and the sequence of stimuli presented was randomized. Stimuli were static greyscale face images (17 cm high) from the NimStim face database [52] and were cropped to remove clothing, background, and hair. This task differed from the one employed by Kyle et al. [24] as follows: different face stimuli, stimulus presentation duration, and response option for intensity ratings was changed from 1–7 to 1–5 as piloting revealed a tendency for participants to not move the hand further along the keyboard to choose higher intensities.

Face-word emotion Stroop task (EST). This task was adapted from the study by Preston and Stansfield [53]. A variable inter-stimulus fixation point was displayed for 500–800 ms before a face of one of three emotions (happy, sad, angry) or neutral expression was displayed for 400 ms. Each face stimuli had the words "happy", "sad", "angry" or "neutral" displayed across the ridge of the nose in order to not obscure facial or eye cues and to appear in the center where the fixation point was previously located. After 400 ms, the stimulus was removed; the task did not proceed to the next trial until the participant responded. The participant responded by indicating the emotion of the face, not the word (using numpad keyboard keys 0–3), as this approximates the original Stroop task where processing of the semantics of the word is automatic and distracting, requiring inhibitory control [54]. There was a total of 36 congruent (face-word matched) and 36 incongruent trials (face-word did not match) for each face type (288 total trials) and the sequence of stimuli presented was randomized. Stimuli were greyscale images (17 cm high) taken from the Karolinska Directed Emotional Faces database [55] and were cropped to remove clothing, background, and hair. This task differed from Preston and Stansfield [53] as follows: different face stimuli, stimulus presentation duration, using the prototypical emotion words ("happy", "sad", "angry") instead of emotion adjectives (e.g., "blissful", "hopeless", "enraged") as the distractor, and the inclusion of a neutral condition ("neutral" word and neutral face expressions).

Sleep recording equipment. Ambulatory PSG was employed using the Prodigy Sleep System (Cerebra Medical Inc., Winnipeg, Canada) in order to capture more naturalistic sleep in participants' homes. The Prodigy Sleep System had eight recording channels: left-frontal EEG and right-frontal EEG, ground and reference, all fixed on the forehead in a box, and drop down electrodes for left EOG, right EOG, right mastoid (M2/A2), and left chin EMG. These channels were used to obtain measures of sleep architecture, average EEG power (μV^2/Hz) for each frequency band over the night, and values of the ORP, a continuous measure of sleep depth ranging 0–2.5 (0 = deepest sleep, 2.5 = awake; [48]).

2.3. Procedure

All the study procedures were cleared by the Brock University Bioscience Research Ethics Board (file#17-322, approval date: 3/28/2018) and the study was conducted in accordance with the Canadian Tri-Council Policy Statement: Ethical Conduct for Research Involving Humans (TCPS2). All subjects gave both verbal and signed consent to participate in the study. For an overview of the study procedure, see Figure 1. Participants were recruited via advertisements on campus and in the community. Individuals interested in the study consented to participation in a preliminary telephone interview to ensure that eligibility criteria were met. Next, they completed a written consent form and additional online questionnaires to further assess eligibility and to collect data on sleep and affect. The subset of the questionnaires reported in the current study included the Pittsburgh Sleep Quality Index (PSQI; [56]) and the Insomnia Severity Index (ISI; [50]), widely used measures of subjective sleep quality, over the past four and two weeks, respectively. The Depression Anxiety Stress Scale (DASS; [57]) and State Trait Anxiety Index–trait (STAI-T; [58]) were completed in order to assess the presence of affective symptomology.

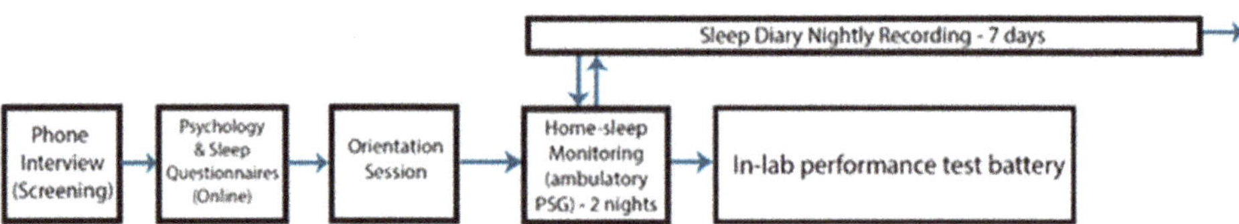

Figure 1. Overview of the progression of study protocol from recruitment to completion.

Eligible participants came to the Sleep Research Laboratory for an orientation session where they signed informed consent for laboratory testing and at-home sleep recording and completed a practice version of the performance assessment battery. They were then instructed on use of the

Prodigy home sleep monitoring equipment which they used for two consecutive nights at home. Additionally, participants completed an online sleep diary following the first night of PSG recording and for up to seven days after. Immediately following the second night of at-home PSG recording, participants came to the lab at 13:00 and had EEG recorded during a performance assessment battery from 14:00 to 16:00. The battery consisted of a number of information processing tasks, not all reported here. In addition to the two emotion processing tasks reported herein, participants also completed a Psychomotor Vigilance Task (PVT), the Stanford Sleepiness Scale (SSS; [59]), the Positive and Negative Affect Schedule (PANAS; [60]), and the STAI-State questionnaire [58], all commonly used to verify changes in waking function due to insufficient sleep. Upon completing the task battery, electrodes were removed and participants were free to leave the lab after debriefing.

2.4. Data Analysis

Sleep files were first scored by automatic sleep-scoring software (Michele software, [61]) following AASM Scoring guidelines [62]. A second pass by a trained human scorer was done to review and edit sleep staging following recommendations from the scoring software. Interclass correlation coefficients between human edited and automatically scored files were calculated for sleep stage times and the coefficient was > 0.8 overall for all files. Sleep scoring yielded the following variables: total sleep time (TST), sleep efficiency (SE), sleep onset latency (SOL), wake after sleep onset (WASO), time in each sleep stage (N1, N2, N3, REM), number of awakenings, total stage shifts, and number of arousals in REM and Non-REM (stages N2 and N3 combined). A discrepancy score between subjective and objective sleep times was calculated for TST, WASO, and SOL, by subtracting PSG values from the sleep diary values for each participant (subjective minus objective). The ORP data as well as average EEG power values for each band were provided by Cerebra Medical Inc on the sleep-scored edited files. EEG measured power was calculated by averaging the squared microvolts of power over the entire sleep file (from lights out to lights on) for each band (delta = 0.33–2.33 Hz, theta = 2.67–6.33 Hz, alpha = 7.33–12 Hz, sigma = 12.33–14.00 Hz, beta-1 = 14.33–20.0 Hz, beta-2 = 20.3–35.00 Hz, beta = average of beta 1 and beta 2) and separately for each EEG channel of the Prodigy equipment: left-frontal and right-frontal EEG channels. Only sleep diary and PSG/EEG data from the second night of recordings which preceded the afternoon of in-lab performance assessment were analyzed.

All variables were tested for violations of normality as well as outliers. Measures violating normality were square-root or log transformed and were tested again for normality. Outliers were identified by box-plots and by individual means greater than +/− 3 SD from the group mean.

Independent sample *t*-tests were used to compare good sleepers and individuals with insomnia symptoms for measures of mood (VAS-M, PANAS, STAI-State), sleepiness (SSS), affect (DASS), anxiety (STAI-Trait), sleep history (ISI, PSQI), sleep architecture, EEG band powers, and ORP values. A two-way ANOVA was conducted for analysis of response time, accuracy and intensity ratings on the Face Categorization and Intensity Rating Task, with between-subjects as Group (GS, INS) and within-subjects as Face (Happy, Sad, Angry, Fearful). For the Face-word Emotion Stroop Task, a three-way ANOVA with the between-subject factor of Group (GS, INS) and within-subject factors of Congruency (congruent, incongruent) and Face (Happy, Sad, Angry, Neutral) was conducted for response times. Equality of variance was examined using Levene's test and violations were corrected using the Welch–Satterthwaite adjustment. For tests of sphericity, violations were corrected using the Greenhouse-Geisser correction.

An exploratory analysis of the interaction between group (GS, INS) and sleep on behavioural performance was conducted using a moderation regression model in PROCESS 3.3 macro for SPSS [63]. For regressions violating heteroscedasticity, heteroscedasticity-consistent standard errors using Hinkley's method [64] were employed in consideration of the small sample size [65]. For the moderation model, predictors were examined independently and included subjective sleepiness, TST, time in Stage 2 sleep, time in SWS, time in REM, ORP Stage 2 sleep, ORP SWS, ORP REM, ORP NREM, PSQI, ISI, and beta power averaged over the two bands (beta-1 and beta-2). The moderation term was group (GS, INS). Further investigation of significant interactions was followed by a simple effects analysis using a bivariate correlational analysis for each group to determine how relationships between sleep and emotion processing outcomes might differ for each group.

Post-hoc Analysis of Poor Sleepers

Because individuals with insomnia do not sleep poorly on every night and previous research has suggested that differences in cognitive functioning occur after a night of poor or short sleep (e.g., [5,6,66]), a secondary post-hoc analysis of sleep and performance on emotion processing tasks was conducted to compare the good sleeper controls to the subset of individuals with insomnia symptoms that were confirmed to have a night of poor sleep prior to performance assessment ($n = 8$). Good and poor nights were judged using multiple variables including TST, SOL, SE, and WASO, from the two nights of PSG recording as well as sleep diary data.

3. Results

3.1. Participant Characteristics

Group comparisons of participant characteristics revealed that the INS group compared to the GS group had significantly greater complaints of insomnia severity and poor historic sleep quality indicated by greater scores on the ISI ($t(18.20) = -6.65$, $p < 0.001$), and PSQI ($t(25) = -11.80$, $p < 0.001$). No differences in affect were observed on the DASS subscales or for STAI-trait (Table 1).

Table 1. Group comparisons and means and standard deviations for historic sleep quality and trait affect.

	Good Sleepers ($n = 14$)		Insomnia ($n = 15$)				
	M	*SD*	*M*	*SD*	*t*	*df*	*Sig. (2-tailed)*
ISI	3.60	2.56	14.21	5.44	−6.65	18.20	**0.001 ****
PSQI	2.87	1.55	11.39	2.14	−12.16	26	**0.001 ****
DASS-Anxiety	2.60	2.29	3.71	4.34	−0.86	19.43	0.403
DASS-Depression	3.73	3.53	6.36	6.78	−1.29	19.28	0.211
DASS-Stress	6.00	4.17	8.71	5.80	−1.46	27	0.157
STAI-Trait	36.87	9.46	39.86	14.07	−0.68	27	0.505

Note. ** = significant at $p < 0.001$.

3.2. Sleep Comparisons by Group

The INS group ($n = 15$) overall reported less TST on the sleep diary ($t(24) = 3.61$, $p < 0.001$), but differences in PSG-measured TST were not observed. No other differences in objective and subjective sleep parameters were observed (Table 2). For quantitative EEG measures of sleep, the INS group did not significantly differ in average power in any band across the night and an examination of group differences in ORP values did not find any differences in sleep depth (Table 3).

Table 2. Group comparisons and means and standard deviations for PSG sleep, sleep diary, and the discrepancy between objective and subjective sleep.

	Good Sleepers ($n = 14$)		Insomnia ($n = 15$)				
	M	*SD*	*M*	*SD*	*t*	*df*	*Sig. (2-tailed)*
	PSG Parameters						
TST	432.82	33.42	393.42	78.27	1.68	15.99	0.113
SE	93.39	2.65	89.74	10.28	1.24	13.48	0.236
SOL	12.39	7.70	16.69	14.79	−0.96	25	0.347
WASO	19.43	10.18	28.08	36.89	−0.82	13.69	0.428
Wake Time	29.83	21.07	40.28	39.20	−0.87	25	0.392

Table 2. Cont.

	Good Sleepers ($n = 14$)		Insomnia ($n = 15$)				
	M	*SD*	*M*	*SD*	*t*	*df*	*Sig. (2-tailed)*
PSG Parameters							
N1 Time	46.94	19.74	42.92	17.84	−0.10	24	0.923
N2 Time	232.90	47.52	203.01	45.81	1.66	25	0.109
N3 Time	80.48	33.76	88.69	30.30	−0.66	25	0.514
REM Time	74.22	18.20	62.42	33.88	1.14	25	0.265
NREM Time	362.65	36.95	336.72	53.71	1.47	25	0.154
Number of Awakenings	16.07	6.04	14.69	7.86	0.51	25	0.612
Total Stage Shifts	129.21	24.95	126.31	35.12	0.25	25	0.805
Number of Arousals in REM	12.36	7.41	12.38	8.09	−0.01	25	0.993
Number of Arousals in Non-REM	73.43	19.64	76.15	33.38	−0.26	19.13	0.801
Sleep Diary							
TST	475.85	50.67	389.23	70.14	3.61	24	**0.001 ***
SOL	12.89	6.60	27.69	35.51	−1.48	12.83	0.163
WASO	6.38	8.20	17.85	20.80	−1.64	11.33	0.128
Sleep Quality Rating (1–7)	4.54	1.51	3.92	0.95	1.24	20.29	0.228
Number of Awakenings	1.92	1.88	3.42	4.42	−1.08	22	0.291
Subject-Objective Discrepancy							
TST	32.38	31.95	−4.19	92.12	1.35	14.85	0.196
SOL	2.08	4.59	11.00	29.18	−1.09	12.59	0.297
WASO	−12.21	12.27	−14.35	43.42	0.20	13.76	0.847

Note. * = significant at $p < 0.05$.

Table 3. Group comparisons and means and standard deviations for quantitative EEG parameters of sleep.

	Good Sleepers ($n = 14$)		Insomnia ($n = 15$)				
Measure	*M*	*SD*	*M*	*SD*	*t*	*df*	*Sig. (2-tailed)*
Average EEG Power							
LF delta	227.26	132.69	208.15	85.48	0.45	26	0.660
RF delta	263.67	153.41	226.53	113.74	0.51	24	0.618
LF theta	13.87	4.78	13.82	3.78	0.03	26	0.975
RF theta	15.58	4.90	15.29	3.82	0.17	24	0.870
LF alpha	5.00	2.60	4.37	1.18	0.80	26	0.430
RF alpha	5.99	2.85	5.08	1.40	1.00	24	0.327
LF sigma	0.71	0.23	0.93	0.45	−1.68	27	0.104
RF sigma	0.85	0.29	1.09	0.49	−1.56	25	0.132
LF beta-1	0.87	0.27	1.04	0.40	−1.36	27	0.186
RF beta-1	0.95	0.30	1.17	0.50	0.51	25	0.181
LF beta-2	0.57	0.36	0.63	0.26	−0.54	27	0.594
RF beta-2	0.60	0.32	0.74	0.44	−1.08	25	0.279
LF beta Average	0.71	0.31	0.84	0.32	−1.10	27	0.277
RF beta Average	0.78	0.30	0.96	0.46	−1.27	25	0.216
ORP Measures							
ORP Non-REM	0.50	0.17	0.51	0.18	−0.23	27	0.905
ORP REM	0.67	0.30	0.74	0.40	−7.08	27	0.638
ORP N1	0.84	0.26	0.89	0.25	−1.06	27	0.609
ORP N2	0.53	0.18	0.54	0.17	−0.33	27	0.869
ORP N3	0.24	0.11	0.25	0.13	−0.18	26	0.883
R/L ORP Correlation	0.87	0.09	0.87	0.12	1.03	26	0.560
ORP Max During Arousal	1.99	0.21	2.00	0.18	−0.38	27	0.925
ORP Baseline Before Arousal	0.63	0.22	0.61	0.21	0.01	27	0.786
Number of Arousals with ORPMax -ORPBaseline > 0.5	45.27	16.95	48.50	26.92	0.66	27	0.886
ORP-9 Post Arousal	0.81	0.20	0.80	0.23	0.03	27	0.700

Note. LF = Left-frontal EEG channel. RF = Right-frontal EEG channel. ORP = Odd Ratio Product (values range from 0 = deepest sleep to 2.5 = wake/arousal).

3.3. State and Psychomotor Vigilance Comparisons by Group

The INS group ($M = 2.64$, $SD = 0.84$) reported being significantly sleepier on the Stanford Sleepiness Scale than the GS ($M = 1.87$, $SD = 0.64$), $t(27) = 2.81$, $p = 0.009$. The INS group ($M = 32.00$, $SD = 8.88$) did not significantly differ from GS ($M = 31.43$, $SD = 5.67$) in positive state affect, nor did the INS group ($M = 12.87$, $SD = 3.56$) differ from GS ($M = 12.79$, $SD = 6.58$) in negative state affect. Further, the INS group ($M = 33.67$, $SD = 7.78$) did not differ in state anxiety from GS ($M = 33.00$, $SD = 6.58$). No evidence for differences between INS and GS groups was observed for psychomotor vigilance performance. Specifically, the INS ($M = 247.16$, $SD = 30.47$) and GS group ($M = 240.81$, $SD = 51.02$) did not differ in response time. There was no difference in number of lapses for the INS group ($M = 0.36$, $SD = 0.50$), compared to GS group ($M = 0.40$, $SD = 0.74$), nor the standard deviation of response time between INS ($M = 51.02$, $SD = 24.24$) and GS groups ($M = 49.40$, $SD = 28.57$). There was no observed difference in average RT for the INS group ($M = 193.65$, $SD = 18.68$) compared to GS ($M = 190.71$, $SD = 19.17$) for the fastest 10% of trials, and no difference in the slowest 10% of trials between INS ($M = 344.26$, $SD = 72.34$) and GS ($M = 330.16$, $SD = 64.94$) groups.

3.4. Emotion Processing Performance: Face-Emotion Categorization and Intensity Rating Task

The descriptive statistics for performance on both emotion tasks by group are presented in Table 4. The results from the analysis for response time, accuracy and intensity rating differences on the FCI are presented as follows:

Table 4. Means and standard deviations for measures from the Face Categorization and Intensity Rating Task (FCI) and the Face-word Emotion Stroop Task (EST).

	Good Sleepers (*n* = 14)		Insomnia (*n* = 15)		All	
	M	*SD*	*M*	*SD*	*M*	*SD*
FCI Response Time						
Happy	402.46	113.92	367.48	92.97	385.57	104.01
Angry	480.93	120.49	448.98	103.10	465.51	103.10
Fearful	496.34	115.62	488.87	87.28	492.73	101.17
Sad	487.78	128.46	460.18	89.03	474.46	110.13
FCI Accuracy						
Happy	0.99	0.01	0.98	0.03	0.98	0.02
Angry	0.90	0.08	0.90	0.08	0.90	0.08
Fearful	0.84	0.12	0.79	0.12	0.82	0.12
Sad	0.86	0.09	0.82	0.13	0.84	0.11
FCI Intensity Ratings						
Happy	2.87	0.49	2.96	0.75	2.91	0.62
Angry	3.30	0.51	3.23	0.48	3.26	0.48
Fearful	3.39	0.48	3.29	0.41	3.34	0.44
Sad	2.92	0.56	2.99	0.55	2.95	0.55
EST Interference (Faces)						
Happy	95.75	58.77	85.15	61.47	90.63	59.25
Angry	126.06	91.91	133.65	86.48	129.73	86.48
Sad	109.55	100.90	119.61	76.94	114.41	88.69
Neutral	137.52	95.87	122.94	101.22	130.48	96.99
EST RT Incongruent Trials (Distractors)						
Happy	1048.60	178.36	1029.85	162.81	1039.55	168.24
Angry	994.90	144.24	977.89	158.19	986.69	148.15
Sad	1000.10	180.46	956.92	148.14	979.25	164.18
Neutral	997.75	207.40	951.96	161.64	975.13	184.82

For response time on the FCI task, the ANOVA revealed a non-significant interaction between Face and Group and no main effect of Group, but there was a significant effect of Face on response time ($F(2.10, 56.78) = 25.95$, $p < 0.001$, $\eta^2 = 0.490$). Happy faces were classified more quickly than Angry ($t(26) = -4.90$, $p < 0.001$), Fearful ($t(26) = -8.10$, $p < 0.001$) and Sad faces ($t(26) = -9.64$, $p < 0.001$).

The Face x Group ANOVA for accuracy yielded a non-significant Face x Group interaction and no main effect of Group, but a significant main effect of Face emotion was observed ($F(1.91, 51.52) = 22.92$, $p < 0.001$, $\eta^2 = 0.459$). Post-hoc comparisons of accuracy of the different expressions revealed that all participants were more accurate for Happy faces than Angry ($t(26) = 6.00$, $p < 0.000$), Fearful ($t(26) = 7.68$, $p < 0.001$), and Sad faces ($t(26) = 7.25$, $p < 0.001$), and more accurate for Angry faces than Fearful faces ($t(26) = 4.72$, $p < 0.001$).

For intensity ratings on the FCI, there was also a significant effect of Face, $F(2.12, 57.11) = 13.75$, $p < 0.001$, $\eta^2 = 0.337$, and again, no significant effect of Group, or significant Group x Face interaction. Post-hoc comparisons between Faces revealed that all participants rated Angry faces as more intense than Happy ($t(26) = 3.20$, $p = 0.020$) and Sad faces ($t(26) = 4.92$, $p < 0.001$), and also rated Fearful faces as more intense than Happy ($t(26) = 4.64$, $p < 0.001$) and Sad faces ($t(26) = 6.60$, $p < 0.001$).

In summary, there were no group differences observed for response time, accuracy and intensity ratings on the FCI. Overall, participants were faster and more accurate for Happy faces compared to other face-types. Additionally, all participants found Angry and Fearful faces as more intense than Happy or Sad faces.

3.5. Emotion Processing Performance: Face-Word Emotion Stroop

For the EST, the three-way interaction for response time was not significant, nor were the two-way interactions of Group x Face, Group x Congruency, or Congruency x Face. There was no main effect of Group. There was a main effect of Congruency on response time, $F(1,27) = 155.31$, $p < 0.001$, $\eta^2 = 0.852$, and post-hoc pairwise comparisons found that all participants were slower for incongruent trials compared to congruent trials, $t = -12.46$, $p < 0.001$. There was also a significant main effect of Face on response time, $F(3,34) = 49.04$, $p < 0.001$, $\eta^2 = 0.879$; post-hoc comparisons revealed that participants were significantly faster for Happy faces compared to Angry ($t(26) = 9.90$, $p < 0.001$), Sad ($t(26) = 9.95$, $p < 0.001$), or Neutral faces ($t(26) = 10.52$, $p < 0.001$). In summary, all participants were slower for incongruent trials compared to congruent trials and were faster for trials with Happy target faces than any other target faces and there were no detectable differences in response times between individuals with INS and GS.

Response time differences for the distractor-words on the EST were also examined. The three-way interaction between Group, Distractor, and Congruency for response times for distractors was non-significant. The two-way interactions between Group and Congruency, and Group and Distractor were also non-significant. There was a significant interaction between Congruency and Distractor for response time on the Emotional Stroop Task, $F(3,81) = 30.80$, $p < 0.001$, $\eta^2 = 0.533$. A post-hoc analysis of distractors at the level of incongruent trials found that all participants were significantly slower for incongruent trials with a Happy distractor than Angry ($t(26) = 4.65$, $p < 0.001$), Neutral ($t(26) = 5.37$, $p < 0.001$) or Sad ($t(26) = 4.53$, $p = 0.001$) distractors (see Table 4). No significant main effect of Group was observed. The distractor word of "Happy" slowed response times more than any other distractors for incongruent trials and the INS group did not differ from GS in response time.

3.6. Post-hoc Analysis of Insomnia Subgroup with a Night of Objectively Poor Sleep

The post-hoc analysis comparing the INS group with a night of poor sleep preceding the afternoon of task performance ($n = 8$) and good sleepers ($n = 15$) revealed that this INS subgroup differed in sleep the night before testing. Specifically, the INS group with a night of poor sleep subjectively reported less total sleep time, $t(19) = 3.77$, $p = 0.001$ and differences in objective sleep architecture were found in less total sleep time ($t(19) = 3.68$, $p = 0.006$), less time in N2 sleep ($t(19) = 2.63$, $p = 0.017$), less time in REM sleep ($t(19) = 2.99$, $p = 0.007$), a smaller portion of time in REM, $t(19) = 2.24$, $p = 0.038$, and less time in Non-REM sleep overall ($t(19) = 3.23$, $p = 0.004$) than GS. This INS subgroup also trended towards greater power in the left-frontal sigma band, $t(21) = -1.96$, $p = 0.064$, and left-frontal beta-1 band, $t(21) = -2.07$, $p = 0.052$, compared to the GS group.

Some evidence for accuracy deficits in the expected direction were observed for this INS subgroup with a night of poor sleep. The ANOVA analysis of FCI accuracy with the INS subgroup with a night of poor sleep ($n = 8$) revealed a trending effect of Group in the direction of the hypothesis (using a 1-tailed test), $F(1,21) = 2.90$, $p = 0.052$, such that the INS group with a night of poor sleep had a trend for poorer accuracy overall on the FCI compared to GS. No other effects were observed in behavioural performance for this post-hoc subgroup analysis.

3.7. Moderation Analysis of Sleep Quality and Emotion Processing by Group

Overall, significant interactions between Group and beta EEG activity and follow up simple slopes analysis found that greater beta EEG activity at frontal sites was associated with greater intensity ratings for emotional faces of Happy, Fearful and Sad (trending), for the insomnia group. For the good sleepers, greater beta EEG activity was associated with poorer accuracy identifying Happy faces, and lower intensity ratings for Happy, Angry, Fearful (trending), and Sad faces. In addition, for good sleepers, greater sleepiness levels were associated with poorer accuracy for Fearful faces, and less time in slow wave sleep was associated with greater intensity ratings of Angry faces. These findings are reported in detail below.

Accuracy. There was a significant interaction between Group and right-frontal beta on accuracy for Happy faces on the FCI, $b = 0.033$, $t = 2.83$, $p = 0.010$. Simple slopes analyses for each Group revealed a significant negative relationship between right-frontal beta and accuracy for Happy faces for good sleepers, $b = -0.02$, $t = -3.99$, $p < 0.001$, but not for the INS group, $b = 0.01$, $t = 1.04$, $p = 0.309$ (Figure 2). For the EST, there was a significant interaction between Group and right-frontal beta on accuracy for incongruent Happy trials, $b = 0.03$, $t = 3.00$, $p = 0.006$. Simple slopes analysis of each Group revealed a significant relationship between greater right-frontal beta power and poorer accuracy for Happy faces on incongruent trials for good sleepers, $b = -0.08$, $t = -3.77$, $p = 0.001$, but no relationship was found for the INS group, $b = 0.00$, $t = 0.01$, $p = 0.996$ (Figure 3). Due to the lower variability in accuracy performance for Happy faces across participants, these relationships are interpreted cautiously.

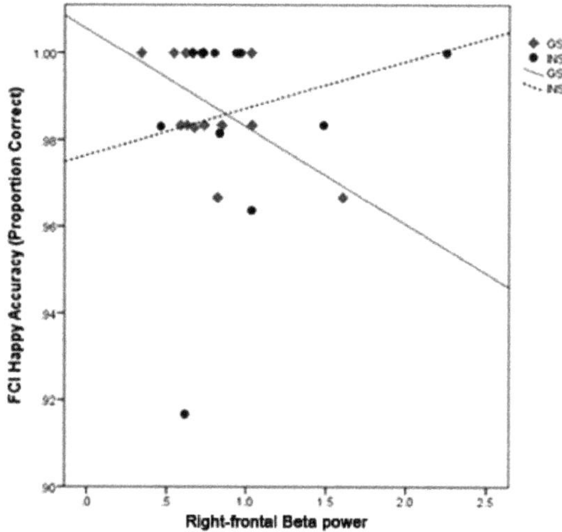

Figure 2. The correlations between right-frontal beta power and accuracy for Happy faces on the FCI for GS and INS groups. A night of greater right-frontal beta activity was associated with lower accuracy for the GS group.

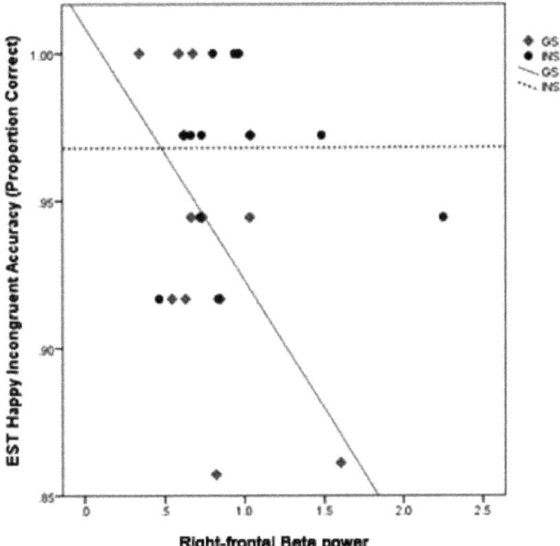

Figure 3. The correlations between right-frontal beta power and accuracy for incongruent Happy face trials on the Emotional-Stroop for GS and INS groups. A night of greater right-frontal beta activity was associated with lower accuracy for Happy faces on incongruent trials for the GS group.

There was a significant interaction between Group and scores on the Stanford Sleepiness Scale on accuracy for Fearful faces on the FCI, $b = 0.15$, $t = 2.89$, $p = 0.008$. The simple effects analysis of each Group found that sleepiness scores were negatively associated with Fearful accuracy for good sleepers, $b = -0.13$, $t = -3.08$, $p = 0.005$, but not significantly associated in the INS group, $b = 0.01$, $t = 0.55$, $p = 0.590$ (Figure 4).

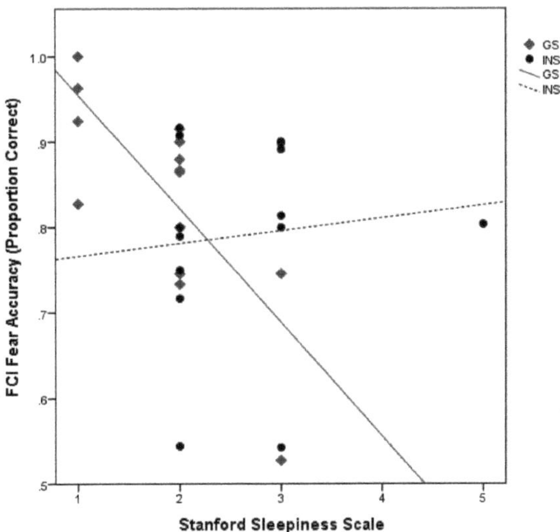

Figure 4. The correlation between Stanford Sleepiness Scale and accuracy for Fearful faces on the FCI for GS and INS groups. Sleepiness levels were negatively associated with Fearful accuracy for GS but not the INS group.

Angry interference. There was significant interaction between Group and right-frontal beta, $b = -283.27$, $t = -4.38$, $p < 0.001$, on the interference effect during Angry trials. The simple slopes analysis for each Group revealed a significant positive correlation between right-frontal beta and Angry interference scores for the good sleepers, $b = 224.40$, $t = 5.31$, $p < 0.001$, but no significant relationship for the INS group, $b = -58.87$, $t = -1.20$, $p = 0.242$ (Figure 5).

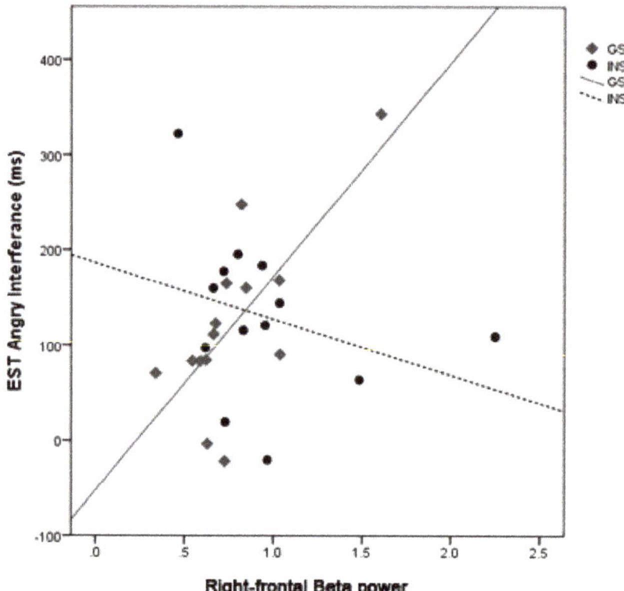

Figure 5. The correlations between right-frontal beta power and the interference effect for Angry trials on the Emotional-Stroop for GS and INS groups. A night of greater right-frontal beta power was associated with greater interference on Angry trials for the GS group.

Intensity ratings. For intensity ratings for Happy faces on the FCI, there was a significant interaction between Group and left-frontal beta power over the night, $b = 1.61$, $t = 4.16$, $p < 0.001$. Simple slopes for each Group revealed a significant negative relationship between left-frontal beta and Happy intensity ratings for good sleepers, $b = -0.47$, $t = -2.32$, $p = 0.029$, but a significant positive relationship for the INS group, $b = 1.13$, $t = -3.46$, $p = 0.002$ (Figure 6). The interaction between Group and right-frontal beta power on intensity ratings for Happy faces was also significant, $b = 1.12$, $t = 3.19$, $p = 0.004$; there was a significant relationship between greater right-frontal beta and greater Happy intensity ratings for the INS group, $b = 0.76$, $t = 4.22$, $p < 0.001$.

There was also a significant interaction between Group and right-frontal beta power on intensity ratings of Angry faces, $b = 0.98$, $t = 3.15$, $p = 0.004$. A simple slopes analysis of each Group revealed a significant relationship between greater right-frontal beta and lower Angry intensity ratings for good sleepers, $b = -0.99$, $t = -3.81$, $p < 0.001$, but no significant relationship was found for the INS group, $b = -0.01$, $t = -0.08$, $p = 0.941$ (see Figure 6). There was also a significant interaction between Group and time in N3 sleep on intensity ratings of Angry faces, $b = 0.01$, $t = 2.97$, $p = 0.007$. A simple slopes analysis for each Group revealed a significant negative relationship between time spent in N3 sleep and Angry face intensity ratings for good sleepers, $b = -0.01$, $t = -2.99$, $p = 0.006$, but no relationship was detected for the INS group, $b = 0.004$, $t = 1.39$, $p = 0.177$.

There was a significant interaction between Group and right-frontal beta on intensity ratings for Fearful faces, $b = 1.09$, $t = 2.97$, $p = 0.007$. The analysis of simple effects for each Group found a significant positive relationship between right-frontal beta and Fearful intensity ratings for the INS group, $b = 0.45$, $t = 6.12$, $p < 0.001$, and a trend for a negative relationship for good sleepers, $b = -0.64$, $t = -1.77$, $p = 0.089$ (Figure 6). There was also a significant interaction between Group and left-frontal beta power on intensity ratings for Fearful faces, $b = 0.96$, $t = 2.33$, $p < 0.028$; analysis for each Group revealed a significant relationship between greater left-frontal beta and greater Fearful intensity ratings for the INS group, $b = 0.67$, $t = 3.40$, $p = 0.002$, but no relationship between these variables for good sleepers, $b = -0.31$, $t = -0.84$, $p = 0.411$.

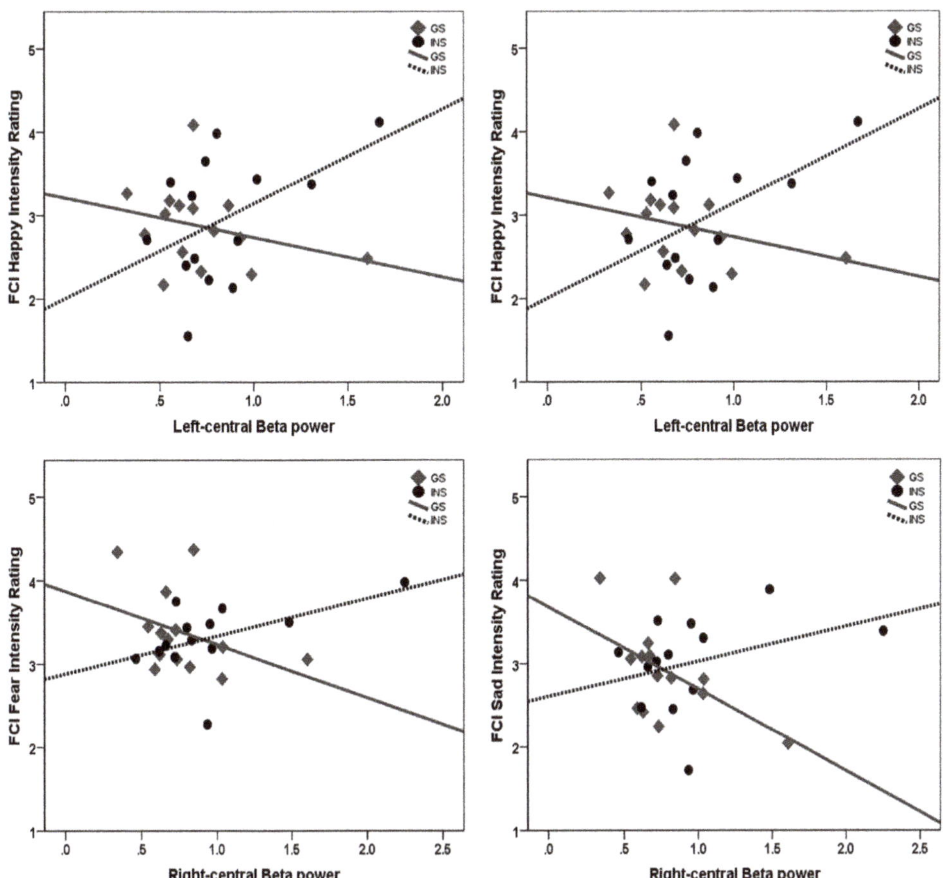

Figure 6. The correlation between frontal beta power and intensity ratings on the FCI for GS and INS groups. Greater frontal beta power was associated with greater intensity ratings of Happy, Fearful and Sad (trending) faces for the INS groups.

Finally, there was a significant interaction between Group and right-frontal beta power on Sad intensity ratings, $b = 0.96$, $t = 2.33$, $p < 0.028$ (Figure 6). The simple slopes analysis for each Group revealed a significant relationship between greater right-frontal beta and lower Sad intensity ratings for good sleepers, $b = -0.98$, $t = -3.03$, $p = 0.006$, but a positive relationship between right-frontal beta and Sad intensity ratings approaching significance for the insomnia group, $b = 0.42$, $t = 2.04$, $p = 0.053$.

4. Discussion

In the current study, emotion processing tasks were examined after a night of PSG recording in order to determine how sleep contributes to next-day processing of emotionally expressive faces in insomnia and good sleepers. The insomnia group was found to be sleepier during the afternoon of performance testing and reported shorter sleep durations than good sleepers despite a lack of evidence for poor sleep quality in PSG measures. Individuals with insomnia did not show any evidence of disturbed mood or affect and no evidence for general impairment in emotion processing performance was found. Greater beta EEG power during the night was associated with greater intensity sensitivity for emotional happy, fearful and a trend for sad faces for individuals with insomnia symptoms. For good sleepers, greater beta EEG power in sleep was associated with poorer perceptual accuracy for happy faces with and without the presence of emotional distractors as well as worse inhibitory control for distracting emotional words when detecting angry faces. In good sleepers, greater beta EEG power was also associated with lower intensity ratings for happy, angry and sad faces and a trend for fearful faces. For the good sleepers but not the insomnia group, greater sleepiness was associated with poorer accuracy for fearful faces, and less time in slow wave sleep was associated with greater sensitivity to angry faces (based on intensity ratings).

4.1. Hyperarousal Differentially Affects Emotion Processing in Good Sleepers and Insomnia

The diverging directions of the relationship between greater frontal beta EEG power during sleep/wake and performance for insomnia and good sleeper groups suggests that hyperarousal (i.e., greater beta EEG power) may be associated with heightened salience processing of emotional face expressions for individuals with insomnia symptoms for some emotions, but in contrast, both blunts sensitivity and leads to emotion processing performance deficits in good sleepers. This points to the possibility for a potential maladaptation or alteration in socioemotional salience processing directly linked to neurophysiological activity at sleep onset and throughout sleep for individuals with insomnia. Possible explanations for these contrasting findings are that for good sleepers, high levels of beta EEG activity may represent a rare night of light, non-restorative sleep (perhaps due to environmental factors), which taxes cognitive resources for next-day functioning. Whereas, for the insomnia group, elevated beta EEG power may represent activity in emotional processing regions throughout sleep that affects next day emotional processing, or alternatively, maladaptation in emotion reactivity during the waking state in insomnia may result in both greater sensitivities to emotional faces and a predisposition for hyperaroused sleep.

Neurophysiological examination of both GABA and regional differences in activity in sleep and wake in insomnia provide evidence that hyperarousal in insomnia may be specific to altered activity in emotion processing regions. GABA is the primary neurotransmitter related to inhibition of the CNS and plays a critical role in sleep initiation, sleep onset and sleep maintenance [67]. Critically, several studies have identified lower GABA levels overall in insomnia [68,69], but one study by Plante and colleagues [70] specifically identified lower levels of morning GABA in the anterior cingulate cortex which is a key structure in emotion information processing including the processing of emotion faces. There has also been imaging evidence for smaller differences in the activity between wake and sleep in regions of affect and face processing, including the left fusiform gyrus and posterior cingulate cortex [22]. Nofzinger and colleagues [71] also found that greater objective or subjective time spent awake throughout the night (i.e., difficulties with sleep maintenance and arousability) were associated with increased activity in the anterior cingulate cortex, and regions associated with emotional awareness, anxiousness and fear (temporal poles). Event-related potential analysis of auditory stimulus processing during sleep for individuals with insomnia has also revealed markers of sustained/uninhibited information processing (e.g., [34,72]). Thus, hyperarousal may represent either the continuous activation or a failure to inhibit the activation of emotional information processing regions during sleep in insomnia, and this may ultimately lead to alterations in the functioning of salience processing during wake. Further research should investigate which regions appear to be active/uninhibited in insomnia sleep to elucidate if hyperarousal or sustained activity exists within emotional regions.

Another possible consideration is that socioemotionally sensitive or reactive individuals are predisposed to nights of hyperarousal. Kalmbach et al. [73] suggested that insomnia may be a condition of dysregulated cognitive-emotional reactivity to stress, ultimately leading to increased reactivity to sleep and thereby, longer periods of sleep onset, greater pre-sleep ruminations and worry, and sleep disruption (i.e., insomnia symptomology). This is not a novel concept, as established models of insomnia have also pointed to maladaptive cognitions and emotion-reactivity, as etiological and pathological qualities of insomnia (see [4] for a review). Intervention with stimulus control and relaxation training for individuals with insomnia has been shown to lead to a reduction in elevated beta EEG activity at sleep-onset [74], supporting the notion that elevated beta may represent maladaptive cognitive-emotional reactivity and conditioned arousal. It is possible that dysregulated or maladaptive cognitive-emotional reactivity in insomnia extends beyond the processing of stressors and negatively conditioned sleep stimuli into the processing of emotional stimuli such as faces as well. A link between hyperarousal and altered waking cognitive-emotional reactivity might be drawn out by EEG examination during wake; increased physiological and subjective arousal during wake in reaction to sleep and non-sleep related emotion stimuli reported in individuals with insomnia [23] has already demonstrated an increase of reactivity to emotion stimuli as a potential feature of this clinical group, but has not been linked to hyperarousal. If hyperarousal in insomnia manifests as a condition of altered cognitive-emotional reactivity during wake, then inconsistent findings in waking hyperarousal [45] may be due to physiological measures predominantly taken while research participants are in resting states rather than in response to emotional stimulation and/or task engagement.

A final possible consideration is that the chronicity and regularity of poor sleep and/or hyperarousal in insomnia might be an important contributing factor to emotion processing differences in insomnia and good sleepers. It has been suggested that sleep plays an integral role in restoring or resetting emotional circuits to correctly react and process emotional information the following day [75]. Thus, repeated nights of poor sleep and/or neurophysiological engagement (hyperarousal insomnia) might disrupt the restorative properties of sleep. In turn, chronic disruption could lead to structural/functional changes in emotional processing neurological regions (e.g., [22,76]) and to abnormal or maladaptive sensitivities to emotional information during wake, beyond that which is seen after a rare night of light or poor sleep in good sleepers. Some evidence suggests that multiple nights of poor sleep is related to greater waking impairment in cognitive functioning (e.g., [8,66]). However, the presence of repeated or consistent nights of hyperaroused sleep in insomnia and the impact that nights of hyperaroused sleep have on waking cognitive functioning has not been well investigated. Nonetheless, several findings of hyperarousal during insomnia sleep [32–42] suggested that it could be a consistent pathological quality of sleep in this clinical population. Therefore, future efforts should be made to longitudinally examine hyperarousal sleep and the impact that it has on waking functioning.

4.2. Sleep and Emotion Processing Group Differences

Except for diary reports of less total sleep time, no significant differences in sleep between good sleepers and individuals with insomnia in the full sample were observed. The finding that individuals with insomnia symptoms subjectively reported less total sleep time than good sleepers in their sleep diaries, despite no observable differences in PSG measure of total sleep time, is consistent with the existing literature (e.g., [77–80]). We identified that eight of the fourteen insomnia participants had a night of poor sleep, while six of the fourteen insomnia participants had a good night of sleep. And, only six of the fourteen individuals with insomnia symptoms reported clinical levels of insomnia on the ISI. Due to the small sample size, all insomnia participants were included together for the primary analyses. Having a small sample, with a mixed and predominantly sub-clinical insomnia group likely affected sensitivity to find the expected group differences in gross sleep architecture, quantitative EEG differences, as well as emotion processing performance. The novel ORP measure (which captures sleep-depth and arousability) may be more suitable to characterizing the sleep of individuals with insomnia that have been specifically identified as having difficulty remaining and/or maintaining sleep and whom have frequent awakenings (i.e., issues with sleep depth and arousability).

In the insomnia group that had a night of poor sleep, we observed a trending effect for greater sigma and beta-1 band power, as well as differences in sleep architecture: less time in Stage 2 and REM sleep. These differences have been previously reported in other studies of sleep in insomnia [31,36,41]. The loss of Stage 2 and REM may be attributable to fewer sleep cycles occurring for those with a night of poor sleep, as both Stage 2 and REM become more prominent later in the night [81]. Greater power in beta and sigma has been suggested to indicate a simultaneous activation of sleep and wake-promoting activity in insomnia sleep [41]. Krystal and colleagues [36] also found elevated sigma and beta activity but only for a subjective phenotype of insomnia and not an objectively poor sleeping insomnia group. Here, we found some evidence for elevated sigma and beta in a small insomnia group objectively identified to have a night of poor sleep.

Two recent reports of impairment in sensitivity for emotionally expressive face stimuli [24,25] for the insomnia group were not replicated here. Kyle and colleagues found individuals with insomnia who had greater anxiety and depressive symptoms had a greater blunting in the intensity ratings of emotional faces [24]. Cronlein and colleagues found impaired accuracy performance for an insomnia group who were identified to have objective nights of poor sleep, but also found similar effects in a group with sleep apnea [25]. Therefore, it is possible that because the current sample failed to show evidence of objective sleep impairment, and participants were recruited based on an absence of affective disturbance (i.e., anxiety or depression), we were unable to detect overall differences in emotion processing performance from good sleepers. It is also possible that some participants with insomnia may show resiliency or compensation with respect to the impact of insufficient sleep on waking performance; these individual differences could be investigated in future research. However, in support of Cronlein and colleague's findings, some evidence for impaired accuracy recognizing faces after a night of poor sleep in insomnia was observed in the current study. In light of the findings by Kyle and colleagues and the current findings of a relationship between beta EEG power during sleep and altered salience processing in insomnia, further research should be conducted on the interplay between hyperarousal during sleep and both affective disturbance and salience processing during wake. It is also suggested that poor sleep in insomnia may lead to performance deficits in emotional face perception, similarly to that which has been reported after nights of experimental sleep deprivation [82–85], which might also contribute to socioemotional impairment. The extent and type of emotional impairment after nights of poor sleep and hyperarousal in insomnia requires further investigation.

4.3. Limitations, Conclusions and Future Directions

The sample was small and included a predominantly subclinical insomnia group with a mixture of good and poor nights of sleep. Thus, the current findings should be interpreted with caution. Future investigations of the effects of sleep (and hyperarousal) in insomnia on waking function must include larger samples to better identify effects, as well as to account for variability in sleep, insomnia subtypes, and the presence or absence of hyperarousal. The sample in the study was also predominantly a convenience sample from the university student body, and as such, the sample was predominantly women and young adults. Therefore, there was no opportunity to examine the effects of sleep and emotion processing between sex, and it is cautioned that any particular effects observed here may be generalizable only to women. Importantly, the findings reported here, or even lack of effects, could be attributable to the skew of more women in the sample, and thus further studies should be done in men. The findings also may not generalize to individuals outside the age range examined for the current study, including older adults for whom insomnia is more prevalent.

Sleep was recorded in participants' own homes in order to increase the ecological validity of the findings which is particularly useful with the insomnia sample who tend to sleep well away from their home environment. However, without strictly enforced bed times, a large portion of the good sleeper participants were lost to sleep restriction, and the insomnia group may have employed strategies such as delaying bedtime which may have contributed to an absence of observable differences in sleep efficiency between groups. In addition, without constant monitoring, some elements of the data, such as data from an EEG channel or sleep diaries, were lost for some participants. A very important limitation to the ambulatory PSG employed in this study was the absence of the ability to detect and rule out sleep apnea and restless leg syndrome. Both conditions were screened for during the intake process by interview and by questionnaire; however, it is possible that participants who are unaware of underlying medical sleep conditions entered the study. Another lack of control in the home environment was that participants could turn the equipment on well before the intention to go to sleep (e.g., reading) despite instruction to record from lights off to on. Thus, measures of wake time, sleep onset latency, and sleep efficiency may not be precise for all participants. Better home monitoring may be achieved with increased controls and measures of compliance as well as an in-lab screening night. A strength of the current study was that performance was assessed on the day immediately following the PSG recording; future studies must endeavour to investigate the impact of the preceding night of sleep on waking performance.

Hyperarousal in the current study was measured by investigating beta EEG during the entire sleep period, including sleep onset, wake time, and non-REM and REM sleep stages together. Higher frequency EEG in the gamma band which has also been associated with hyperarousal was not investigated in the current study because of hardware filters imposed on the data, but should be examined in future studies. In addition, the beta EEG reported in the current study was not separated by wake and sleep stages. While some studies have reported hyperarousal specific to stages of sleep [36,38,41], others have noted the presence of hyperarousal in pre-sleep wake and at sleep onset as well (during the effortful intention to fall asleep; [74,86,87], and some during both pre-sleep wake and sleep [35,42]. Because we had a heterogeneous sample of individuals with insomnia symptoms (i.e., not exclusively sleep onset or maintenance problems), we choose to sample the entire sleep/wake record for EEG analysis. Since groups did not differ in wake time, it is likely that at least some of the elevated beta EEG is coming from sleep, although future studies in larger samples of more homogenous insomnia subtypes may be able to better address the hyperarousal during wake and sleep states (or even transitions and arousals).

This study investigated the relationship between quantitative EEG measures of sleep and the next-day socioemotional processing of faces in individuals with insomnia symptoms and good sleepers. The contrasting associations between beta EEG activity and emotion processing for good sleepers and insomnia groups suggests that hyperarousal in insomnia may lead to waking consequences of altered salience processing, and more specifically, to heightened sensitivity to emotionally expressive faces. Given the limitations of the sample, further studies are warranted. The following research questions are recommended to be addressed by future research efforts: are emotion processing areas engaged during hyperarousal sleep; are the same areas engaged during hyperarousal in both good sleepers and individuals with insomnia; does hyperarousal have functional significance for good sleepers as well; finally, is hyperarousal associated with abnormal neurophysiological reactivity to emotional cues during wake? Clinically, the findings suggest that hyperarousal in insomnia relates to abnormal sensitivity to emotionally expressive faces, which could contribute to the reported experiences of poorer social functioning. Interventions which restore or curtail neurophysiological activity during sleep to normative levels may also serve to improve socioemotional functioning by restoring appropriate sensitivity to the emotional expressions of others. Further confirmation of the impact of hyperarousal and a night of poor sleep on emotion processing in insomnia could also inform possible treatments or inventions for the development of comorbid social deficiencies, anxiety and/or depression.

Author Contributions: Conceptualization, R.D.M.H. and K.A.C.; methodology, R.D.M.H., K.A.C., K.J.M., K.A.L.; validation, K.J.M.; formal analysis, R.D.M.H., K.A.C., K.J.M., K.A.L.; investigation, R.D.M.H.; data curation, R.D.M.H.; writing—original draft preparation, R.D.M.H., K.A.C.; writing—review and editing, R.D.M.H., K.A.C., K.J.M., K.A.L.; supervision, K.A.C.; project administration, K.A.C.; funding acquisition, K.A.C. All authors have read and agreed to the published version of the manuscript.

Funding: This work was supported by institutional research seed grants, including the Council for Research in Social Sciences (CRISS) from the Faculty of Social Sciences at Brock University, the Brock University Advancement Fund (BUAF), and by the Brock Library Open Access Publishing Fund.

Acknowledgments: Thank you to Magdy Younus and Mark Younus for providing EEG analysis of sleep data from Prodigy sleep recorder and the inter-class correlation analysis on sleep scoring.

Conflicts of Interest: The authors declare no conflict of interest.

References

1. Morin, C.M.; Leblanc, M.; Bélanger, L.; Ivers, H.; Mérette, C.; Savard, J. Prevalence of insomnia and its treatment in Canada. *Can. J. Psychiatry* **2011**, *56*, 540–548. [CrossRef] [PubMed]
2. Morin, C.M.; LeBlanc, M.; Daley, M.; Gregoire, J.P.; Mérette, C. Epidemiology of insomnia: Prevalence, self-help treatments, consultations, and determinants of help-seeking behaviors. *Sleep Med.* **2006**, *7*, 123–130. [CrossRef] [PubMed]
3. Pallesen, S.; Sivertsen, B.; Nordhus, I.H.; Bjorvatn, B. A 10-year trend of insomnia prevalence in the adult Norwegian population. *Sleep Med.* **2014**, *15*, 173–179. [CrossRef] [PubMed]
4. Perlis, M.L.; Ellis, J.G.; Kloss, J.D.; Riemann, D.W. Etiology and pathophysiology of insomnia. In *Principles and Practice of Sleep Medicine*, 6th ed.; Kryger, M., Roth, T., Dement, W., Eds.; Elesvier: Amsterdam, The Netherlands, 2017; pp. 769–784.
5. Bastien, C.H.; Fortier-Brochu, É.; Rioux, I.; LeBlanc, M.; Daley, M.; Morin, C.M. Cognitive performance and sleep quality in the elderly suffering from chronic insomnia: Relationship between objective and subjective measures. *J. Psychosom. Res.* **2003**, *54*, 39–49. [CrossRef]
6. Fernandez-Mendoza, J.; Calhoun, S.; Bixler, E.O.; Pejovic, S.; Karataraki, M.; Liao, D.; Vela-Bueno, A.; Ramos-Platon, M.J.; Sauder, K.A.; Vgontzas, A.N. Insomnia with objective short sleep duration is associated with deficits in neuropsychological performance: A general population study. *Sleep* **2010**, *33*, 459–465. [CrossRef]
7. Ferrie, J.E.; Shipley, M.J.; Akbaraly, T.N.; Marmot, M.G.; Kivimäki, M.; Singh-Manoux, A. Change in sleep duration and cognitive function: Findings from the Whitehall II Study. *Sleep* **2011**, *34*, 565–573.
8. Fortier-Brochu, E.; Morin, C.M. Cognitive impairment in individuals with insomnia: Clinical significance and correlates. *Sleep* **2014**, *37*, 1787–1798. [CrossRef]
9. Li, Y.; Liu, H.; Weed, J.G.; Ren, R.; Sun, Y.; Tan, L.; Tang, X. Deficits in attention performance are associated with insufficiency of slow-wave sleep in insomnia. *Sleep Med.* **2016**, *24*, 124–130. [CrossRef]
10. Shekleton, J.A.; Flynn-Evans, E.E.; Miller, B.; Epstein, L.J.; Kirsch, D.; Brogna, L.A.; Burke, L.M.; Bremer, E.; Murray, J.M.; Gehrman, P.; et al. Neurobehavioral performance impairment in insomnia: Relationships with self-reported sleep and daytime functioning. *Sleep* **2014**, *37*, 107–116. [CrossRef]
11. Wardle-Pinkston, S.; Slavish, D.C.; Taylor, D.J. Insomnia and cognitive performance: A systematic review and meta-analysis. *Sleep Med. Rev.* **2019**, *48*, 101205. [CrossRef]
12. Carey, T.J.; Moul, D.E.; Pilkonis, P.; Germain, A.; Buysse, D.J. Focusing on the experience of insomnia. *Behav. Sleep Med.* **2005**, *3*, 73–86. [CrossRef] [PubMed]
13. Endeshaw, Y.W.; Yoo, W. Association between social and physical activities and insomnia symptoms among community-dwelling older adults. *J. Aging Health* **2016**, *28*, 1073–1089. [PubMed]
14. Silva, J.A.; Chase, M.; Sartorius, N.; Roth, T. Special report from a symposium held by the world health organization and the world federation of sleep research societies. *Overview Insomnias Rel. Disord.—Recog.* **1996**, *19*, 412–416.
15. Kyle, S.D.; Crawford, M.R.; Morgan, K.; Spiegelhalder, K.; Clark, A.A.; Espie, C.A. The Glasgow Sleep Impact Index (GSII): A novel patient-centred measure for assessing sleep-related quality of life impairment in Insomnia Disorder. *Sleep Med.* **2013**, *14*, 493–501. [CrossRef]
16. Cote, K.; Lustig, K.; MacDonald, K. The role of sleep in processing emotional information. In *Handbook of Sleep Research*; Dringenberg, H., Ed.; Academic Press: Cambridge, MA, USA, 2019; Volume 30.
17. Beattie, L.; Kyle, S.D.; Espie, C.A.; Biello, S.M. Social interactions, emotion and sleep: A systematic review and research agenda. *Sleep Med. Rev.* **2015**, *24*, 83–100.

18. Baglioni, C.; Spiegelhalder, K.; Regen, W.; Feige, B.; Nissen, C.; Lombardo, C.; Violani, C.; Hennig, J.; Riemann, D. Insomnia disorder is associated with increased amygdala reactivity to insomnia-related stimuli. *Sleep* **2014**, *37*, 1907–1917.

19. Li, C.; Ma, X.; Dong, M.; Yin, Y.; Hua, K.; Li, M.; Li, C.; Zhan, W.; Li, C.; Jiang, G. Abnormal spontaneous regional brain activity in primary insomnia: A resting-state functional magnetic resonance imaging study. *Neuropsychiatr. Dis. Treat.* **2016**, *12*, 1371–1378.

20. Dai, X.J.; Peng, D.C.; Gong, H.H.; Wan, A.L.; Nie, X.; Li, H.J.; Wang, Y.X. Altered intrinsic regional brain spontaneous activity and subjective sleep quality in patients with chronic primary insomnia: A resting-state fMRI study. *Neuropsychiatr. Dis. Treat.* **2014**, *10*, 2163–2175. [CrossRef]

21. Kay, D.B.; Karim, H.T.; Soehner, A.M.; Hasler, B.P.; James, J.A.; Germain, A.; Hall, M.H.; Franzen, P.L.; Price, J.C.; Nofzinger, E.A.; et al. Subjective–Objective sleep discrepancy is associated with alterations in regional glucose metabolism in patients with insomnia and good sleeper controls. *Sleep* **2017**, *40*, zsx155.

22. Kay, D.B.; Karim, H.T.; Soehner, A.M.; Hasler, B.P.; Wilckens, K.A.; James, J.A.; Aizenstein, H.J.; Price, J.C.; Rosario, B.L.; Kupfer, D.J.; et al. Sleep-wake differences in relative regional cerebral metabolic rate for glucose among patients with insomnia compared with good sleepers. *Sleep* **2016**, *39*, 1779–1794.

23. Baglioni, C.; Lombardo, C.; Bux, E.; Hansen, S.; Salveta, C.; Biello, S.; Violani, C.; Espie, C.A. Psychophysiological reactivity to sleep-related emotional stimuli in primary insomnia. *Behav. Res. Ther.* **2010**, *48*, 467–475. [CrossRef] [PubMed]

24. Kyle, S.D.; Beattie, L.; Spiegelhalder, K.; Rogers, Z.; Espie, C.A. Altered emotion perception in insomnia disorder. *Sleep* **2014**, *37*, 775–783. [CrossRef] [PubMed]

25. Crönlein, T.; Langguth, B.; Eichhammer, P.; Busch, V. Impaired recognition of facially expressed emotions in different groups of patients with sleep disorders. *PLoS ONE* **2016**, *11*, e0152754. [CrossRef] [PubMed]

26. Blair, R.J. Facial expressions, their communicatory functions and neuro–cognitive substrates. *Philos. Trans. R. Soc. Lond. Ser. B Biol. Sci.* **2003**, *358*, 561–572. [CrossRef] [PubMed]

27. Hess, U.; Fischer, A. Emotional mimicry as social regulation. *Personal. Soc. Psychol. Rev.* **2013**, *17*, 142–157. [CrossRef] [PubMed]

28. Marsh, A.A.; Blair, R.J. Deficits in facial affect recognition among antisocial populations: A meta-analysis. *Neurosci. Biobehav. Rev.* **2007**, *32*, 454–465. [CrossRef]

29. Kushida, C.A.; Littner, M.R.; Morgenthaler, T.; Alessi, C.A.; Bailey, D.; Coleman, J., Jr.; Friedman, L.; Hirshkowitz, M.; Kapen, S.; Kramer, M.; et al. Practice parameters for the indications for polysomnography and related procedures: An update for 2005. *Sleep* **2005**, *28*, 499–523. [CrossRef]

30. Edinger, J.D.; Ulmer, C.S.; Means, M.K. Sensitivity and specificity of polysomnographic criteria for defining insomnia. *J. Clin. Sleep Med.* **2013**, *9*, 481–491. [CrossRef]

31. Baglioni, C.; Regen, W.; Teghen, A.; Spiegelhalder, K.; Feige, B.; Nissen, C.; Riemann, D. Sleep changes in the disorder of insomnia: A meta-analysis of polysomnographic studies. *Sleep Med. Rev.* **2014**, *18*, 195–213. [CrossRef]

32. Buysse, D.J.; Germain, A.; Hall, M.L.; Moul, D.E.; Nofzinger, E.A.; Begley, A.; Ehlers, C.L.; Thompson, W.; Kupfer, D.J. EEG spectral analysis in primary insomnia: NREM period effects and sex differences. *Sleep* **2008**, *31*, 1673–1682. [CrossRef]

33. Bastien, C.H.; Turcotte, I.; St-Jean, G.; Morin, C.M.; Carrier, J. Information processing varies between insomnia types: Measures of N1 and P2 during the night. *Behav. Sleep Med.* **2013**, *11*, 56–72. [CrossRef] [PubMed]

34. Ceklic, T.; Bastien, C.H. Information processing during NREM sleep and sleep quality in insomnia. *Int. J. Psychophysiol.* **2015**, *98*, 460–469. [CrossRef] [PubMed]

35. Fernandez-Mendoza, J.; Li, Y.; Vgontzas, A.N.; Fang, J.; Gaines, J.; Calhoun, S.L.; Liao, D.; Bixler, E.O. Insomnia is associated with cortical hyperarousal as early as adolescence. *Sleep* **2016**, *39*, 1029–1036. [CrossRef] [PubMed]

36. Krystal, A.D.; Edinger, J.D.; Wohlgemuth, W.K.; Marsh, G.R. NREM sleep EEG frequency spectral correlates of sleep complaints in primary insomnia subtypes. *Sleep* **2002**, *25*, 626–636.

37. Merica, H.; Blois, R.; Gaillard, J.M. Spectral characteristics of sleep EEG in chronic insomnia. *Eur. J. Neurosci.* **1998**, *10*, 1826–1834. [CrossRef]

38. Perlis, M.L.; Smith, M.T.; Andrews, P.J.; Orff, H.; Giles, D.E. Beta/Gamma EEG activity in patients with primary and secondary insomnia and good sleeper controls. *Sleep* **2001**, *24*, 110–117. [CrossRef]

39. Perlis, M.L.; Giles, D.E.; Mendelson, W.B.; Bootzin, R.R.; Wyatt, J.K. Psychophysiological insomnia: The behavioural model and a neurocognitive perspective. *J. Sleep Res.* **1997**, *6*, 179–188. [CrossRef]

40. Riedner, B.A.; Goldstein, M.R.; Plante, D.T.; Rumble, M.E.; Ferrarelli, F.; Tononi, G.; Benca, R.M. Regional patterns of elevated alpha and high-frequency electroencephalographic activity during nonrapid eye movement sleep in chronic insomnia: A pilot study. *Sleep* **2016**, *39*, 801–812. [CrossRef]

41. Spiegelhalder, K.; Regen, W.; Feige, B.; Holz, J.; Piosczyk, H.; Baglioni, C.; Riemann, D.; Nissen, C. Increased EEG sigma and beta power during NREM sleep in primary insomnia. *Biol. Psychol.* **2012**, *91*, 329–333. [CrossRef]

42. Freedman, R.R. EEG power spectra in sleep-onset insomnia. *Electroencephalogr. Clin. Neurophysiol.* **1986**, *63*, 408–413. [CrossRef]

43. Schomer, D.L.; Lopes da Silva, F.H. *Nidermeyer's Electroencephalography: Basic Principles, Clinical Applications, and Related Fields*, 7th ed.; Oxford University Press: Oxford, UK, 2017.

44. Bonnet, M.H.; Arand, D.L. Hyperarousal and insomnia: State of the science. *Sleep Med. Rev.* **2010**, *14*, 9–15. [CrossRef] [PubMed]

45. Kay, D.B.; Buysse, D.J. Hyperarousal and beyond: New insights to the pathophysiology of insomnia disorder through functional neuroimaging studies. *Brain Sci.* **2017**, *7*, 23. [CrossRef] [PubMed]

46. Riemann, D.; Spiegelhalder, K.; Feige, B.; Voderholzer, U.; Berger, M.; Perlis, M.; Nissen, C. The hyperarousal model of insomnia: A review of the concept and its evidence. *Sleep Med. Rev.* **2010**, *14*, 19–31. [CrossRef] [PubMed]

47. Wilckens, K.A.; Woo, S.G.; Kirk, A.R.; Erickson, K.I.; Wheeler, M.E. Role of sleep continuity and total sleep time in executive function across the adult lifespan. *Psychol. Aging* **2014**, *29*, 658–665. [CrossRef]

48. Younes, M.; Ostrowski, M.; Soiferman, M.; Younes, H.; Younes, M.; Raneri, J.; Hanly, P. Odds ratio product of sleep EEG as a continuous measure of sleep state. *Sleep* **2015**, *38*, 641–654. [CrossRef]

49. American Psychiatric Association. *Diagnostic and Statistical Manual of Mental Disorders*, 5th ed.; Author: Arlington, VA, USA, 2013.

50. Morin, C.M.; Belleville, G.; Bélanger, L.; Ivers, H. The insomnia severity index: Psychometric indicators to detect insomnia cases and evaluate treatment response. *Sleep* **2011**, *34*, 601–608. [CrossRef]

51. Morin, C.M. *Relief from Insomnia*; Doubleday/Dell: New York, NY, USA, 1996.

52. Tottenham, N.; Tanaka, J.W.; Leon, A.C.; McCarry, T.; Nurse, M.; Hare, T.A.; Marcus, D.J.; Westerlund, A.; Casey, B.J.; Nelson, C. The NimStim set of facial expressions: Judgments from untrained research participants. *Psychiatry Res.* **2009**, *168*, 242–249. [CrossRef]

53. Preston, S.D.; Stansfield, R.B. I know how you feel: Task-irrelevant facial expressions are spontaneously processed at a semantic level. *Cogn. Affect. Behav. Neurosci.* **2008**, *8*, 54–64. [CrossRef]

54. Stroop, J.R. Studies of interference in serial verbal reactions. *J. Exp. Psychol.* **1935**, *18*, 643–662. [CrossRef]

55. Lundwist, D.; Flykt, A.; Ohman, A. *The Karolinska Directed Emotional Faces-KDEF*; Department of Clinical Neuro-science, Psychology section, Karolinska Institutet: Stockholm, Sweden, 1998.

56. Buysse, D.J.; Reynolds, C.F.; Monk, T.H.; Berman, S.R.; Kupfer, D.J. The Pittsburgh sleep quality index: A new instrument for psychiatric practice and research. *Psychiatry Res.* **1989**, *28*, 193–213. [CrossRef]

57. Lovibond, S.H.; Lovibond, P.F. *Manual for the Depression Anxiety & Stress Scales*, 2nd ed.; Psychology Foundation: Sydney, Australia, 1995.

58. Spielberger, C.D. State-Trait anxiety inventory. In *The Corsini Encyclopedia of Psychology*; John Wiley & Sons, Inc.: Hoboken, NJ, USA, 2010.

59. Hoddes, E.; Zarcone, V.; Dement, W. Stanford Sleepiness Scale. In *Enzyklopädie der Schlafmedizin*; Springer: Berlin/Heidelberg, Germany, 2007; p. 1184.

60. Watson, D.; Clark, L.A.; Tellegen, A. Development and validation of brief measures of positive and negative affect: The PANAS scales. *J. Personal. Soc. Psychol.* **1988**, *54*, 1063–1070. [CrossRef]

61. Malhotra, A.; Younes, M.; Kuna, S.T.; Benca, R.; Kushida, C.A.; Walsh, J.; Hanlon, A.; Staley, B.; Pack, A.I.; Pien, G.W. Performance of an automated polysomnography scoring system versus computer-assisted manual scoring. *Sleep* **2013**, *36*, 573–582. [CrossRef]

62. Berry, R.B.; Brooks, R.; Gamaldo, C.E.; Harding, S.M.; Marcus, C.L.; Vaughn, B.V. *The AASM Manual for the Scoring of Sleep and Associated Events*; American Academy of Sleep Medicine: Darien, IL, USA, 2012.

63. Hayes, A.F. PROCESS: A Versatile Computational Tool for Observed Variable Mediation, Moderation, and Conditional Process modeling. Available online: https://www.afhayes.com/public/process2012.pdf (accessed on 15 June 2019).

64. Hinkley, D.V. Jackknifing in unbalanced situations. *Technometrics* **1977**, *19*, 285–292. [CrossRef]

65. Hayes, A.F.; Cai, L. Using heteroskedasticity-consistent standard error estimators in OLS regression: An introduction and software implementation. *Behav. Res. Methods* **2007**, *39*, 709–722. [CrossRef] [PubMed]

66. Hansen, D.A.; Layton, M.E.; Riedy, S.M.; Van Dongen, H.P. Psychomotor vigilance impairment during total sleep deprivation is exacerbated in sleep-onset insomnia. *Nat. Sci. Sleep* **2019**, *11*, 401–410. [CrossRef] [PubMed]

67. Gottesmann, C. GABA mechanisms and sleep. *Neuroscience* **2002**, *111*, 231–239. [CrossRef]

68. Winkelman, J.W.; Buxton, O.M.; Jensen, J.E.; Benson, K.L.; O'Connor, S.P.; Wang, W.; Renshaw, P.F. Reduced brain GABA in primary insomnia: Preliminary data from 4T proton magnetic resonance spectroscopy (1H-MRS). *Sleep* **2008**, *31*, 1499–1506. [CrossRef]

69. Klumpp, H.; Post, D.; Angstadt, M.; Fitzgerald, D.A.; Phan, K.L. Anterior cingulate cortex and insula response during indirect and direct processing of emotional faces in generalized social anxiety disorder. *Biol. Mood Anxiety Disord.* **2013**, *3*, 7. [CrossRef]

70. Plante, D.T.; Jensen, J.E.; Schoerning, L.; Winkelman, J.W. Reduced γ-aminobutyric acid in occipital and anterior cingulate cortices in primary insomnia: A link to major depressive disorder? *Neuropsychopharmacology* **2012**, *37*, 1548–1557. [CrossRef]

71. Nofzinger, E.A.; Nissen, C.; Germain, A.; Moul, D.; Hall, M.; Price, J.C.; Buysse, D.J. Regional cerebral metabolic correlates of WASO during NREM sleep in insomnia. *J. Clin. Sleep Med.* **2006**, *2*, 316–322. [CrossRef]

72. Kertesz, R.S.; Cote, K.A. Event-related potentials reveal failure to inhibit stimuli during the pre-sleep waking period for patients with sleep-onset insomnia. *Behav. Sleep Med.* **2011**, *9*, 68–85. [CrossRef] [PubMed]

73. Kalmbach, D.A.; Anderson, J.R.; Drake, C.L. The impact of stress on sleep: Pathogenic sleep reactivity as a vulnerability to insomnia and circadian disorders. *J. Sleep Res.* **2018**, *27*, e12710. [CrossRef] [PubMed]

74. Jacobs, G.D.; Benson, H.; Friedman, R. Home-based central nervous system assessment of a multifactor behavioral intervention for chronic sleep-onset insomnia. *Behav. Ther.* **1993**, *24*, 159–174. [CrossRef]

75. Walker, M.P.; van Der Helm, E. Overnight therapy? The role of sleep in emotional brain processing. *Psychol. Bull.* **2009**, *135*, 731–748. [CrossRef]

76. Zhao, L.; Wang, E.; Zhang, X.; Karama, S.; Khundrakpam, B.; Zhang, H.; Guan, M.; Wang, M.; Cheng, J.; Shi, D.; et al. Cortical structural connectivity alterations in primary insomnia: Insights from MRI-based morphometric correlation analysis. *Biomed Res. Int.* 2015. [CrossRef]

77. Frankel, B.L.; Coursey, R.D.; Buchbinder, R.; Snyder, F. Recorded and reported sleep in chronic primary insomnia. *Arch. Gen. Psychiatry* **1976**, *33*, 615–623. [CrossRef]

78. Reite, M.; Buysse, D.; Reynolds, C.; Mendelson, W. The use of polysomnography in the evaluation of insomnia. *Sleep* **1995**, *18*, 58–70. [CrossRef]

79. Spinweber, C.L.; Johnson, L.C.; Chin, L.A. Disqualified and qualified poor sleepers: Subjective and objective variables. *Health Psychol.* **1985**, *4*, 569–578. [CrossRef]

80. Edinger, J.D.; Fins, A.I.; Glenn, D.M.; Sullivan, R.J., Jr.; Bastian, L.A.; Marsh, G.R.; Dailey, D.; Hope, T.V.; Young, M.; Shaw, E.; et al. Insomnia and the eye of the beholder: Are there clinical markers of objective sleep disturbances among adults with and without insomnia complaints? *J. Consult. Clin. Psychol.* **2000**, *68*, 586. [CrossRef]

81. Carskadon, M.A.; Dement, W.C. Normal Human Sleep: An Overview. In *Principles and Practice of Sleep Medicine*, 6th ed.; Kryger, M., Roth, T., Dement, W., Eds.; Elsevier: Amsterdam, The Netherlands, 2017; pp. 15–24.

82. Cote, K.; Mondloch, C.; Sergeeva, V.; Taylor, M.; Semplonius, T. Impact of total sleep deprivation on behavioural neural processing of emotionally expressive faces. *Exp. Brain Res.* **2014**, *232*, 1429–1442. [CrossRef]

83. Killgore, W.B.; Balkin, T.J.; Yarnell, A.M.; Capaldi, V.F. Sleep deprivation impairs recognition of specific emotions. *Neurobiol. Sleep Circadian Rhythm.* **2017**, *3*, 10–16. [CrossRef] [PubMed]

84. Maccari, L.; Martella, D.; Marotta, A.; Sebastiani, M.; Banaj, N.; Fuentes, L.J.; Casagrande, M. Effects of sleep loss on emotion recognition: A dissociation between face and word stimuli. *Exp. Brain Res.* **2014**, *232*, 3147–3157. [CrossRef] [PubMed]
85. Van Der Helm, E.; Gujar, N.; Walker, M.P. Sleep deprivation impairs the accurate recognition of human emotions. *Sleep* **2010**, *33*, 335–342. [CrossRef] [PubMed]
86. Lamarche, C.H.; Ogilvie, R.D. Electrophysiological changes during the sleep onset period of psychophysiological insomniacs. Psychiatric insomniacs, and normal sleepers. *Sleep* **1997**, *20*, 726–733. [CrossRef]
87. Staner, L.; Cornette, F.; Maurice, D.; Viardot, G.; Bon, O.L.; Haba, J.; Staner, C.; Luthringer, R.; Muzet, A.; Macher, J.P. Sleep microstructure around sleep onset differentiates major depressive insomnia from primary insomnia. *J. Sleep Res.* **2003**, *12*, 319–330. [CrossRef]

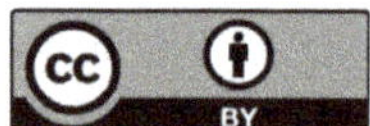

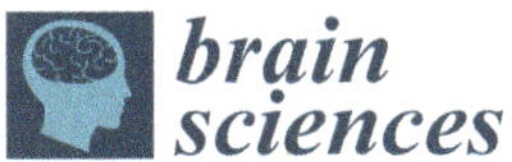

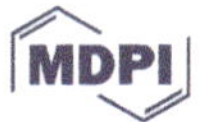

Article

Driving After Drinking Alcohol Associated with Insufficient Sleep and Insomnia among Student Athletes and Non-Athletes

Celyne H. Bastien [1,*], Jason G. Ellis [2], Amy Athey [3], Subhajit Chakravorty [4], Rebecca Robbins [5], Adam P. Knowlden [6], Jonathan Charest [1] and Michael A. Grandner [7]

[1] School of Psychology, Laval University, Quebec, QC G1V0A6, Canada; jonathan.charest.2@ulaval.ca
[2] Northumbria Sleep Research Laboratory, Northumbria University, Newcastle-Upon-Tyne NE1 8ST, UK; jason.ellis@northumbria.ac.uk
[3] Department of Athletics, University of Arizona, Tucson, AZ 85721, USA; athey@email.arizona.edu
[4] Departments of R & D Psychiatry, Corporal Michael J. Crescenz VA Medical Center, Perelman School of Medicine, Philadelphia, PA 19104, USA; Subhajit.Chakravorty@uphs.upenn.edu
[5] Department of Population Health, NYU School of Medicine, New York, NY 10016, USA; Rebecca.Robbins@nyumc.org
[6] Department of Health Science, University of Alabama, Tuscaloosa, AL 35401, USA; aknowlden@ches.ua.edu
[7] Psychiatry, Psychology, and Medicine, University of Arizona College of Medicine, Tucson, AZ 85713, USA; grandner@email.arizona.edu
* Correspondence: celyne.bastien@psy.ulaval.ca; Tel.: +1-418-656-2131 (ext. 8344)

Received: 29 January 2019; Accepted: 18 February 2019; Published: 20 February 2019

Abstract: Introduction: The proportion of university/college students (UCS) consuming alcohol is similar to the number of those reporting poor sleep, at approximately 30%, the proportion being greater in student athletes (SA). What remains to be understood is if poor sleep potentiates risky behaviors. Objective: Our aim was to examine the association among sleep difficulties, insomnia symptoms, and insufficient sleep on the risk of driving under the influence of alcohol in a sample of UCS and whether these associations were more pertinent in SA. Methods: Data from the National University/College Health Assessment was used from the years 2011–2014. Questions on number of drinks consumed and behaviors such as driving after drinking alcohol were related to answers to questions pertaining to sleep difficulties, insufficient sleep, and insomnia symptoms. Results: Mean alcohol intake was of about 3 drinks; SA consumed significantly more than student non-athletes (SNA). Binge-drinking episodes were significantly higher among SA than SNA. Difficulty sleeping was associated with an increased likelihood of driving after any drinks and after 5 or more drinks in both groups, effects being stronger among SA. Insomnia was associated with an increased likelihood of driving after any drinks and after 5 or more drinks in SA and after 5 or more drinks in SNA. These effects were stronger among athletes. Conclusion: The present study found that self-reported difficulties sleeping, insomnia symptoms, and insufficient sleep are associated with driving after drinking alcohol. This relationship applied to driving after drinking any alcohol or binge drinking and was again stronger among SA than SNA.

Keywords: students; athletes; driving after drinking alcohol; insufficient sleep; insomnia

---

1. Introduction

University/college student (UCS) alcohol consumption and poor sleep habits are prominent public health concerns due to their endemic prevalence and their association with multiple negative health outcomes [1,2]. Nearly 60% of full-time UCS consume alcohol [3], with an estimated 37.9% engaging in binge drinking [4]. Alcohol intake is a leading cause of injury in UCS, implicated in

1825 deaths per year [5]. Nationally, 28.9% of UCS reported operating a motor vehicle while under the influence of alcohol in the past month, and 10.5% were injured because of drinking [5]. More specifically for students, alcohol use is also associated with numerous academic consequences, including missed classes, performing poorly on examinations, and overall lower grades [6].

Sleep among adolescents has been linked to adverse outcomes regarding school performance. Lund and colleagues [7] identified 60% of UCS in their sample as having poor sleep quality on the Pittsburgh Sleep Quality Index (PSQI) and found higher reported alcohol intake within this group. Insufficient sleep duration of less than 7 h (defined based on recommendations from the American Academy of Sleep Medicine and Sleep Research Society [8] and National Sleep Foundation [9]) has also been suggested to increase the risk of unintentional injury and impede academic performance [10]. Identifying associations between alcohol consumption and sleep difficulties is especially concerning among UCS as this population reports worse sleep quality than the general population [7,11]. Typically, students present an irregular sleep/wake cycle [12] in addition to insufficient sleep and decreased sleep quality, with those parameters negatively influencing cognitive and psychological processes. Insufficient sleep also affects attention and school performance (academia) [13–15], increases risky behaviors [16], and perturbs social relationships [17]. An altered quality of sleep has also been shown to directly affect health by increasing anxiety [18], depressive thoughts and suicide ideations [15], and diminishes general health quality [19].

Interestingly, it is estimated that approximately 60% of UCS consumed alcohol in the preceding month [20], which is similar to the 60% reporting poor sleep quality noted above [7]. Similar prevalence rates and associated risk of unintentional injury, particularly within the realm of risky driving behaviors, imply a possible association between alcohol consumption and poor sleep in UCS. The relation between risky behaviors, especially driving after alcohol use and with sleep complaints in adolescents and young adults, is still understudied. However, results from a recent survey in high school students (50,370) showed that not sleeping the recommended number of hours during school days (9 h in this case), led to increased risky behaviors, which included drinking and driving [21]. More than 90% of the students reported an insufficient sleep duration during an average school night. Similarly, Wong, Robertson and Dyson [22] recently observed that the risk of driving under the influence of alcohol in adolescents, as well as other risky behaviors including drug-use problems, could be predicted within one year by sleep difficulties, and especially by reports of difficulties getting off to sleep/staying asleep and insufficient sleep. Specifically, trouble failing asleep positively predicted the odds of binge drinking and driving while drunk [22]. Recent studies are attempting to identify neural mechanisms underlying repercussions of short and poor sleep quality on emotional processes in adolescents [23]. One longitudinal study assessed annually insomnia symptoms in early adolescent girls aged 9 to 13 years, and 3 years later, they measured the neural reward processing through fMRI [24]. It was found that self-reported poor sleep quality was positively associated with the dorsal medial prefrontal cortex (DMPFC) response to reward anticipation [24]. Moreover, sleep deprivation amplifies amygdala reactivity in response to negative stimuli, associated with a loss of prefrontal cortex connectivity [25]. This lack of connectivity increases the phenomena of maladaptive interpretation of pleasure [26–28]. Alcohol has been shown to cause an increase of dopamine in the reward pathway [29]. The dopamine in the reward pathway is suggested to increases craving for alcohol and reinforces habitual alcohol use [30]. Thus, SA who are sleep deprived may be oblivious to the fact that their dopamine level will lead them into drinking more alcohol.

Student athletes (SA) may face particularly steep barriers to sleep compared to Students non-athletes (SNA). Barriers to sleep among SA include balancing school demands, sport performance, training, and traveling for competitions (often creating jet-lag and sleeping in different locations than their own bed) (National Collegiate Athletic Association (NCAA), 2014) [31]. Leeder, Glaister, Pizzoferro, Dawson, & Pedlar [32] have shown, using actigraphy, that objective sleep quality is worse in SA than in SNA, including longer sleep-onset latencies, increased time in bed, and time awake after-sleep-onset, more fragmented sleep, and decreased sleep efficiencies. Furthermore, one study revealed that SA were more prone to daytime sleepiness than SNA [33]. Survey data derived from the NCAA [31] revealed that SA report, on average, four poor nights of sleep per week, albeit insufficient sleep, insomnia symptoms, or difficulty sleeping.

The aim of the present research was to further examine the associations among sleep difficulties, insomnia symptoms and insufficient sleep on the risk of driving under the influence of alcohol in a sample of UCS. Because sleep problems appear to be linked to risky behavior in adolescents, it should also be the case in UCS, an at-risk group who are at the transition between adolescence and adulthood. In addition, because SA report even greater sleep difficulties than SNA [32], this association might be stronger in athletes than in SNA and so this was also examined. Because insomnia symptoms and insufficient sleep are significant sleep difficulties observed in UCS, it was predicted that increasing insomnia symptoms and insufficient sleep would be closely related to driving after drinking alcohol.

2. Methods

2.1. Data Source

Data from the National University/college Health Assessment (NCHA) was used. The NCHA is an annual survey conducted by the American university/College Health Association (ACHA) [34] to document the prevalence and changes in a wide range of health-related factors among UCS. This survey provides the largest known data source on health factors among American university/college and UCS. Surveys were administered on paper or online. Survey data from 2011–2014 were used, as items did not change during this time period. Data were obtained from 44, 51, 57, and 34 universities/colleges in 2011, 2012, 2013, and 2014, respectively (though for the sake of de-identifying responses, more information about the institutions is not available). This resulted in data from $N = 27{,}774$ in 2011, $N = 28{,}237$ in 2012, $N = 32{,}964$ in 2013, and $N = 25{,}841$ in 2014. Varsity athletes were identified by self-report, though no information was available regarding sport played or division of the NCAA, the governing body of collegiate athletics. Of note, NCAA division describes the level of competition (I being most competitive, III being less competitive). Since analyses were secondary to a de-identified data set, the project was exempted from the institutional review board oversight, because as an archival analysis of de-identified data, it is not human subject research.

2.2. Measures

"Difficulty Sleeping" was assessed with the item, "Within the past 12 months, have any of the following been traumatic or very difficult for you to handle?" One of the listed conditions was "Sleep Difficulties." This was recorded as "Yes" or "No." Insomnia symptoms were assessed with the item, "In the last 7 days, how often have you had an extremely hard time falling asleep?" Difficulty Initiating Sleep (DIS) was coded "Yes" if the participant noted difficulty falling asleep 3 or more nights per week, consistent with research diagnostic criteria [35]. Of note, this reflects insomnia symptomology, but does not include chronicity nor associated impairment so it cannot alone reflect "insomnia." Perceived insufficient sleep was assessed with the item, "On how many of the past 7 days did you get enough sleep so that you felt rested when you woke up in the morning?" This variable was coded as a continuous variable, recoded so that values reflected nights of insufficient sleep (e.g., individuals who reported 7 nights of sufficient rest were given a score of 0 nights of insufficient sleep). Of note, this may or may not reflect short sleep duration, but rather perceived insufficiency. This is similar to variables used in previous studies [36–38].

Alcohol intake was assessed with the item, "The last time you "partied"/socialized, how many drinks of alcohol did you have?" This was assessed as a continuous variable. Binge drinking was assessed as, "Over the last 2 weeks, how many times have you had five or more drinks of alcohol at a sitting?" This was also assessed as a continuous variable.

Any driving was assessed with the items, "Within the last 30 days, did you drive after drinking any alcohol at all?" and binge drinking was evaluated with the question "Within the last 30 days, did you drive after drinking five or more drinks of alcohol?" Responses were coded as "Yes" or "No." Subjects who reported that they did not drink or did not drive at all in the past 30 days were excluded from analysis.

Status as a student athlete was determined based on the item, "Within the last 12 months, have you participated in organized university/college athletics at any of the following levels?" Students were considered SA (SA) if they indicated "Varsity Sports" and SNA if they did not (those indicating "Club Sports" or "Intramurals" were still considered SNA). Age and sex, which were self-reported, as well as survey year were the covariates in this analysis.

2.3. Statistical Analyses

All variables were assessed using descriptive statistics (mean and standard deviation for continuous variables and percentages for categorical variables). Overall differences between SA and SNA were evaluated with T-tests and Chi-Square tests. To determine whether athlete status interacts with sleep variables on drinking and driving, binomial logistic regression analyses were used, with drinking and driving as outcome variables (both "any drinks" and "5 or more drinks"), age, sex, and survey year as covariates, sleep variable (difficulty sleeping, DIS, and insufficient sleep) as predictor variable and an interaction term for each sleep variable by student athlete status. If this interaction term was significant, further analyses were stratified by student athlete status. These stratified analyses would include drinking and driving variables (separately) as outcome, sleep variables (separately) as predictors, and age, sex, and survey year as covariates. Post-hoc analyses examined whether results were mediated by DIS or alcohol, by including the DIS variable as an additional covariate or adding both number of drinks and binge-drinking episodes as an additional covariate. p values < 0.05 were categorized as statistically significant, though all p values are reported. All analyses were performed using STATA 14.0 (STATA Corp., University/college Station, TX, USA).

3. Results

3.1. Characteristics of the Sample

Sample characteristics are reported in Table 1. The sample consisted of UCSs sampled between 2011–2014. Of the total sample, approximately 8% were varsity athletes. When SA and SNA were compared (also displayed in Table 1), SNA were older than SA (t (111, 496) = 50.66, p < 0.001). Chi-squares analyses showed that the sample comprised more women than men, $\chi^2(2) = 111.59$, p > 0.05, both groups being composed of more women than men while proportionally more men were SA than SNA. Mean alcohol intake during the last socializing period was a mean of about 3.2 drinks (SD = 3.8); SA consumed significantly more than SNA. Number of binge episodes was also significantly higher among SA, compared to SNA (see Table 1).

When SA and SNA were asked if they had driven under the influence of alcohol, athletes were less likely to say yes than SNA when their alcohol consumption was less than 5 drinks (any drinks). However, groups provided similar answers to the same question for 5 drinks and more. Chi-square analyses showed that SNA were more likely to report difficulty sleeping and DIS than SA (χ^2 respectively of 168.70 and 33.49; p < 0.0001). Also, SNA were more likely to report insufficient sleep than SA (t (111, 496) = 4.90, p < 0.001). Thus, SA are generally less likely to report sleep disturbances than SNA. Finally, because this survey was completed over 4 years, chi-square analyses revealed that 2013 and 2014 were different on the percentage of individuals completing the survey per year. As such, proportionally more SA individuals completed the survey in 2013 than on 2014, years 2011 and 2012 being equal on the percentage of individuals completing the survey.

Table 1. Characteristics of the Sample.

Variable	Description	Complete Sample	Student Non-Athlete	Student Athlete	Test Statistic	p
N		111,498	102,815	8683		
Age	Years	21.5 ± 3.6	21.7 ± 3.7	19.6 ± 1.9	50.66	<0.0001
Gender	Female	66.63%	67.07%	61.49%	110.59	<0.0001
Number of Drinks Consumed	Drinks	3.18 ± 3.78	3.10 ± 3.69	3.92 ± 4.45	-19.49	<0.0001
Binge-Drinking Episodes	Episodes	0.73 ± 1.46	0.71 ± 1.43	0.95 ± 1.60	-14.71	<0.0001
Driving after any drinking	Yes	23.95%	24.83%	13.68%	344.24	<0.0001
Driving after binge drinking	Yes	2.48%	2.46%	2.67%	0.88	0.3485
Sleep difficulties	Yes	25.68%	26.17%	19.81%	168.70	<0.0001
Difficulty Initiating Sleep	Yes	24.35%	24.57%	21.78%	33.49	<0.0001
Insufficient sleep	Days per week	3.93 ± 1.91	3.94 ± 1.92	3.84 ± 1.86	4.90	<0.0001
Survey year	2011	24.33%	24.20%	25.94%	109.31	<0.0001
	2012	24.42%	24.23%	26.70%		
	2013	28.53%	28.49%	29.01%		
	2014	22.71%	23.08%	18.36%		

3.2. Driving Under the Influence of Alcohol and Difficulty Sleeping

A significant interaction between difficulty sleeping and athletics status was found (see Table 2). In stratified analyses (Table 3), difficulty sleeping was associated with an increased likelihood of driving after any drinks and after 5 or more drinks in both groups, but the effects were stronger among SA. Overall, SNA who reported a difficulty sleeping were 1% more likely to drive after any drinks and 51% more likely to drive after 5 or more drinks, compared to those without difficulties. In comparison, SA with a difficulty sleeping were 42% more likely to drive after any drinks and 112% more likely to drive after 5 or more drinks, compared to those without difficulty sleeping. All driving variables were associated with difficulty sleeping even after adjusting for the effects of age, sex, and survey years.

Table 2. Athlete Status by Sleep Interactions on Driving After Drinking Alcohol, With and Without Adjustment for Amount of Drinking.

Interaction	Interaction Chi-Square (Without Drinking)	p	Interaction Chi-Square (With Drinking)	p
Outcome: Driving after Any Drinking Any Drinks				
Sleep Difficulty	123.41	<0.0001	138.24	<0.0001
Difficulty Initiating Sleep	106.10	<0.0001	143.95	<0.0001
Insufficient Sleep	106.88	<0.0001	198.32	<0.0001
Outcome: Driving after Binge Drinking at Least 5 Drinks				
Sleep Difficulty	72.42	<0.0001	34.67	<0.0001
Difficulty Initiating Sleep	28.17	<0.0001	6.02	0.110
Insufficient Sleep	18.73	0.0003	23.42	0.076

Table 3. Associations between Driving After Drinking Alcohol and Sleep Variables in Student Athletes and Non-Athletes.

	Non-Athlete					Athlete			
Driving After Drinking	Sleep Variable	OR	95% CI	p	Driving After Drinking	Sleep Variable	OR	95% CI	p
Model 1: Adjusted for Age, Sex, and Survey Year									
Any drinking	Sleep Difficulty	1.008	(1.033–1.123)	0.0005 **	Any drinking	Sleep Difficulty	1.416	(1.169–1.716)	0.0003 **
Binge drinking	Sleep Difficulty	1.511	(1.355–1.686)	<0.0001 **	Binge drinking	Sleep Difficulty	2.123	(1.452–3.104)	0.0001 **
Any drinking	Insufficient Sleep	1.005	(0.995–1.015)	0.2954	Any drinking	Insufficient Sleep	1.052	(1.006–1.100)	0.0275 *
Binge drinking	Insufficient Sleep	1.077	(1.047–1.107)	<0.0001 **	Binge drinking	Insufficient Sleep	1.106	(1.004–1.218)	0.0419 *
Any drinking	Difficulty Initiating Sleep	0.987	(0.945–1.031)	0.5482	Any drinking	Difficulty Initiating Sleep	1.318	(1.091–1.593)	0.0041 *
Binge drinking	Difficulty Initiating Sleep	1.262	(1.125–1.415)	<0.0001 **	Binge drinking	Difficulty Initiating Sleep	1.935	(1.325–2.825)	0.0006 **
Model 2: Adjusted for Age, Sex, Survey Year, and Difficulty Initiating Sleep									
Any drinking	Sleep Difficulty	1.096	(1.047–1.147)	<0.0001 **	Any drinking	Sleep Difficulty	1.316	(1.068–1.620)	0.0097 *
Binge drinking	Sleep Difficulty	1.43	(1.297–1.650)	<0.0001 **	Binge drinking	Sleep Difficulty	1.762	(1.158–2.681)	0.0081 *
Any drinking	Insufficient Sleep	1.006	(0.996–1.017)	0.2162	Any drinking	Insufficient Sleep	1.042	(0.995–1.091)	0.083
Binge drinking	Insufficient Sleep	1.069	(1.039–1.099)	<0.0001 **	Binge drinking	Insufficient Sleep	1.081	(0.978–1.195)	0.1289
Model 3: Adjusted for Age, Sex, Survey Year, Number of Drinks, and Binge Drinking									
Any Drinking	Sleep Difficulty	1.027	(0.984–1.072)	0.214	Any Drinking	Sleep Difficulty	1.306	(1.072–1.591)	0.008 *
Binge Drinking	Sleep Difficulty	1.348	(1.203–1.510)	<0.0001 **	Binge Drinking	Sleep Difficulty	1.779	(1.197–2.644)	0.004 *
Any Drinking	Insufficient Sleep	0.996	(0.986–1.006)	0.451	Any Drinking	Insufficient Sleep	1.032	(0.986–1.081)	0.177
Binge Drinking	Insufficient Sleep	1.051	(1.022–1.082)	0.001 **	Binge Drinking	Insufficient Sleep	1.070	(0.968–1.182)	0.187
Any Drinking	Difficulty Initiating Sleep	0.927	(0.886–0.969)	0.001 **	Any Drinking	Difficulty Initiating Sleep	1.189	(0.980–1.445)	0.080
Binge Drinking	Difficulty Initiating Sleep	1.040	(0.922–1.172)	0.526	Binge Drinking	Difficulty Initiating Sleep	1.654	(1.117–2.451)	0.012 *

Table 3 Caption: Results displayed as Odds Ratio (OR) and 95% Confidence Interval (95% CI). The total number of analyses was 3 (sleep variables) × 2 (drinking outcomes) × 2 (athlete status), or 12 tests for models 1 and 3, and 8 tests for model 2 (due to inclusion of difficulty initiating sleep as a covariate). This yields a total of 32 tests. If a Bonferroni correction were applied based on this number of tests, the new significance criterion would be 0.0015. Please note that in Table 3, * = significant at 0.05 and ** = significant at 0.0015.

3.3. Driving Under the Influence of Alcohol and Insufficient Sleep

A significant interaction between insufficient sleep and athlete status was found (see Table 2). In stratified analyses (Table 3), insufficient sleep was not associated with an increased likelihood of driving after any drinks in SNA, but all other comparisons were significant. Effects were again stronger among athletes. Thus, SNA with insufficient sleep were 1% more likely to drive after any drinks and 8% more likely to drive after 5 or more drinks per day of insufficient sleep. On the other hand, SA were 5% more likely to drive after any drinks and 11% more likely to drive after 5 or more drinks for each day of insufficient sleep that they report.

3.4. Driving Under the Influence of Alcohol and DIS

A significant interaction between DIS and athletics was found (see Table 2). In stratified analyses (Table 3), controlling for age, gender, and survey year, DIS was associated with an increased likelihood of driving after any drinks and after 5 or more drinks in SA and after 5 or more drinks in SNA. Once more, effects were stronger among athletes. SNA with DIS were less than 1% more likely to drive after any drinks and 26% more likely to drive after 5 or more drinks, compared to those without DIS. In comparison, SA with DIS were 32% more likely to drive after any drinks and 93% more likely to drive after 5 or more drinks, compared to SA without DIS.

3.5. Driving Under the Influence of Alcohol while Controlling for DIS

After controlling for DIS (Table 3), in addition to controlling for age, gender, and survey year, a difficulty sleeping was associated with an increased likelihood of driving after any drinks and after 5 or more drinks in both groups, but the effects were even stronger among athletes than among SNA. It appeared that SNA with a difficulty sleeping were 10% more likely to drive after any drinks and 43% more likely to drive after 5 or more drinks, compared to those without difficulties. Conversely, SA with a difficulty sleeping were 32% more likely to drive after any drinks and 76% more likely to drive after 5 or more drinks, compared to SA without a difficulty sleeping.

After controlling for age, gender, survey year and DIS, insufficient sleep was also associated with an increased likelihood of driving after any drinks and after 5 or more drinks in SA and after more than 5 drinks in SNA. Effects were again somewhat stronger among athletes than in SNA. Altogether, SNA with insufficient sleep were 1% more likely to drive after any drinks and 7% more likely to drive after 5 or more drinks, per day of insufficient sleep. On the other hand, for each day that SA reported sleep, they were 4% more likely to drive after any drinks and 8% more likely to drive after 5 or more drinks.

3.6. Driving Under the Influence of Alcohol while Controlling for Amount of Drinking

Finally, after controlling for drinking as well as age, sex, and survey year, a difficulty sleeping was associated with an increased likelihood of driving after any drinks in SA only, though when analyses were examined for binge drinking, results were significant for both groups, though the effect was nominally larger among SA. Insufficient sleep was no longer associated with driving after drinking alcohol in either group, except that was associated with driving after binge drinking in SNA only. DIS was still associated with driving after any drinks, but only in SNA, and DIS was still associated with driving after binge drinking, but only in SA.

4. Discussion

This research examined the association between sleep difficulties, DIS, and insufficient sleep in UCS and drinking behavior. Furthermore, it assessed whether a sleeping difficulty, insufficient sleep, and DIS potentiated drinking and driving behavior in SA vs. SNA. Our results indicate that not only does DIS and insufficient sleep significantly increase the likelihood of drinking and driving (especially for 5 or more drinks), difficulty sleeping was also associated with drinking and driving. Furthermore, it appears that the association between driving under the influence of alcohol and DIS/insufficient sleep is stronger among athletes than non-athletes.

Our study found that SA drank more alcohol and reported fewer sleep disturbances, compared to SNA. They were also less likely to drive after any drinking, and there was no difference in rates of driving after binge drinking. These findings provide a context for the interactive effects that were examined as the primary analyses in this study. Previous studies have shown that SA drink more alcohol [39], and the present study supports this. Large studies of student athlete sleep are not available, but existing evidence suggests that rates of sleep disturbances are quite high among SA [32], as well as students in general [7] though rates of sleep disturbances may not be much different and may even favor SNA.

It is possible that athletes, who typically have a more regular schedule, may experience fewer sleep problems than SNA. Although no differences were seen in rates of driving after binge drinking (rare in both athletes and SNA), driving after drinking any alcohol was less common among athletes. This may reflect increased access to transportation, concerns about getting in trouble and not being able to play, awareness of their high visibility in the community, or increased access to educational interventions.

Among both SA and SNA, sleep difficulties were associated with increased likelihood of driving after consuming alcohol. This may be related to emotional dysregulation as a common upstream factor. Students using alcohol as a mean to cope with stressful situations do expose themselves to greater alcohol consumption and thus to sleep difficulties [40,41]. Therefore, worse mental health may predispose one to problem drinking and sleep difficulties, as well as poor decision-making (leading to driving after drinking). There are several other plausible reasons why these are related. Sleep disturbances have been repeatedly shown to be related to both affective dysregulation [42] (which can lead to excessive drinking) and poor decision-making [43] (which can lead to driving after drinking). Alcohol consumption also leads to both sleep disturbances [44] and poor decision-making [45]. It seems likely that sleep difficulties, alcohol consumption, and impaired decision-making may all be inter-related, leading to this relationship.

There is also evidence that hormones can have different influence on behavior during puberty and adulthood. For example, a tendency toward increased risk taking and sensation seeking may represent a set of normative developmental changes in adolescence [46]. Another strong evidence that supports a link between increases level of hormone and puberty is demonstrated through several studies [47,48]. These data are in line with an anthropological perspective on risk taking in adolescent which can be viewed as an adaptive willingness to establish bravery to acquire a better social status. These findings support the idea that SA may be more prone to peer and status-sensitive influences on risky decision-making as explained by Steinberg [49].

This relationship was stronger, though, among athletes. It is possible that the increased alcohol consumption increased the incapacitated decision-making process. Perhaps the natures of the drinking or sleep disturbances are fundamentally different, leading to a different relationship. Also, it may have to do with social pressure. SA are more likely to be more widely known (for example, in their respective institution or even at a country level) than non-SA. Being recognized by others in a public place where alcohol is served may well lead to peer pressure (cannot refuse offers) and add to the overall 'culture' of alcohol consumption among students, athletes or not, which is then established. In that sense, it has been shown that athletes even expect to receive free alcoholic beverages from peers [50]. This may well reinforce a culture that supports heavy drinking in this population [51]. Thus, it is plausible to assume that they will behave in a manner consistent with accepted drinking patterns of the peers in their immediate environment [52]. However, it is difficult to assert which problem comes first. Are sleep difficulties in athletes conducive to drinking and then ultimately driving under the influence or is the alcohol causing the sleep difficulties? Among UCS, individuals reporting poor sleep quality tend to drink more frequently and excessively [7,40,53], it is our suggestion that sleep difficulties need to be addressed as a priority, considering the benefits of good sleep on the health and general risky behavior in students. In fact, the motivations for drinking, as elegantly stated by Digdon and colleagues [54] may be particularly influential for sleep-deprived students who may experience impaired physical and executive functioning in high-risk drinking contexts. Sleep-deprived students may lack alternative means for managing affect, as a result. Thus, SA may be more prone again to engage in heavy alcohol consumption than SNA.

Limitations

There are several limitations to the current study. First, the sleep items included in the questionnaire were not extracted from validated sleep questionnaires. Thus, their reliability and validity have not been rigorously ascertained. With that in mind, results should be interpreted with a certain degree of caution. Second, the cross-sectional nature of the study precludes any inferences of causality. It may be the case that poor sleep leads to drinking and driving, or it may be the case that factors that contribute to this behavior similarly cause sleep disturbances. A further possibility is that sleep loss may lead to poor decision-making, which itself may lead to poor sleep (directly and indirectly through increased drinking). Third, there is no objective verification of driving after drinking, and therefore the rates are likely underreported. Fourth, it is unknown whether athletes were Division I, II, or III, which may play a role in athletic, academic, and/or social factors.

5. Conclusions

The present study found that a self-reported difficulty sleeping, DIS, and insufficient sleep are associated with driving after drinking alcohol. This relationship applied to driving after any alcohol, and driving after binge drinking. This relationship was stronger among SA than it was for non-SA. These results suggest that sleep disturbances are an independent risk factor for the activity of driving after drinking alcohol. Future research should aim to determine whether driving after drinking alcohol could be reduced by improving sleep health. Also, more clarity on the specific contributions of sleep, measured using validated and/or objective methods, would aid in the interpretation of these results.

Author Contributions: Conceptualization, C.H.B.; Data curation, M.A.G.; Formal analysis, C.H.B. and M.A.G.; Funding acquisition, M.A.G.; Writing—original draft, C.H.B.; Writing—review & editing, J.G.E., A.A., S.C., R.R., A.P.K., J.C. and M.A.G.

Acknowledgments: C.H.B. would like to acknowledge the financial support of the University Laval; A.A. of University of Arizona Department of Athletics; S.C. of a VA grant IK2CX000855 and MAG, 5K23HL110216 and a NCAA Innovations in Research & Practice grant.

Conflicts of Interest: The authors declare no conflict of interest.

References

1. Weshler, H.; Nelson, T.B. What We Have Learned from the Harvard School of Public Health College Alcohol Study: Focusing Attention on College Student Alcohol Consumption and the Environmental Conditions That Promote It. *J. Stud. Alcohol Drugs* **2008**, *69*, 1–10.
2. Hershner, S.D.; Chervin, R.D. Causes and consequences of sleepiness among college students. *Nat. Sci. Sleep* **2014**, *6*, 73–84. [CrossRef]
3. Lipari, R.N.; Jean-Francois, B. A Day in the Life of College Students Aged 18 to 22: Substance Use Facts. *The CBHSQ Report. Rockville (MD): Substance Abuse and Mental Health Services Administration (US)*; 26 May 2016. Available online: https://www.ncbi.nlm.nih.gov/books/NBK396154/ (accessed on 1 November 2018).
4. National Survey from the Substance Abuse and Mental Health Services Administration. Mental Health Services: Rockville, MD, USA, 2015. Available online: https://samhda.s3-us-gov-west-1.amazonaws.com/s3fs-public/field-uploads-protected/studies/NSDUH-2015/NSDUH-2015-datasets/NSDUH-2015-DS0001/NSDUH-2015-DS0001-info/NSDUH-2015-DS0001-info-codebook.pdf (accessed on 1 November 2018).
5. Hingson, R.W.; Zha, W.; Weitzman, E.R. Magnitude of and Trends in Alcohol-Related Mortality and Morbidity Among U.S. College Students Ages 18–24, 1998–2005. *J. Stud. Alcohol Drugs Suppl.* **2009**, *16*, 12–20. [CrossRef]

6.   Weshler, H.; Nelson, T.B. Binge drinking and the American College Student: What's five drinks? *Psychol. Addict. Behav.* **2001**, *15*, 287–291.

7.   Lund, H.G.; Reider, B.D.; Whiting, A.B.; Prichard, J.R. Sleep patterns and predictors of disturbed sleep in a large population of university/college students. *J. Adolesc. Health* **2010**, *46*, 124–132. [CrossRef] [PubMed]

8.   Watson, N.F.; Badr, M.S.; Belenky, G.; Bliwise, D.L.; Buxton, O.M.; Buysse, D.; Dinges, D.F.; Gangwisch, J.; Grandner, M.A.; Kushida, C.; et al. Recommended amount of sleep for a healthy adult: A joint consensus statement of the American Academy of Sleep Medicine and Sleep Research Society. *Sleep* **2015**, *38*, 843–844. [CrossRef] [PubMed]

9.   Hirshkowitz, M.; Whiton, K.; Albert, S.M.; Alessi, C.; Bruni, O.; DonCarlos, L.; Hazen, N.; Herman, J.; Adams Hillard, P.J.; Katz, E.S.; et al. National sleep Foundation's updated sleep duration recommendations: Final report. *Sleep Health* **2015**, *1*, 233–243. [CrossRef]

10.   Taylor, D.J.; Bramoweth, A.D. Patterns and consequences of inadequate sleep in college students: Substance use and motor vehicle accidents. *J. Adolesc. Health* **2010**, *46*, 610–612. [CrossRef]

11.   Forquer, L.M.; Camden, A.E.; Gabriau, K.M.; Johnson, C.M. Sleep patterns of university/college students at a public university/college. *J. Am. Coll. Health* **2008**, *56*, 563–565. [CrossRef]

12.   Wittmann, M.; Dinich, J.; Merrow, M.; Roenneberg, T. Social jetlag: Misalignment of biological and social time. *Chronobiol. Int.* **2006**, *23*, 497–509. [CrossRef]

13.   Dewald, J.F.; Meijer, A.M.; Oort, F.J.; Kerkhof, G.A.; Bogels, S.M. The influence of sleep quality, sleep duration and sleepiness on school performance in children and adolescents: A meta-analytic review. *Sleep Med. Rev.* **2010**, *14*, 179–189. [CrossRef] [PubMed]

14.   Gaultney, J.F. The prevalence of sleep disorders in university/college students: Impact on academic performance. *J. Am. Coll. Health* **2010**, *59*, 91–97. [CrossRef] [PubMed]

15.   Owens, J.; Adolescent Sleep Working Group; Committee on Adolescence. Insufficient sleep in adolescents and young adults: An update on causes and consequences. *Pediatrics* **2014**, *134*, e921–e932. [CrossRef] [PubMed]

16.   Womack, S.D.; Hook, J.N.; Reyna, S.H.; Ramos, M. Sleep loss and risk-taking behavior: A review of the literature. *Behav. Sleep Med.* **2013**, *11*, 343–359. [CrossRef] [PubMed]

17.   Gordon, A.M.; Chen, S. The role of sleep in interpersonal conflict: Do sleepless nights mean worse fights? *Soc. Psychol. Personal. Sci.* **2014**, *5*, 168–175. [CrossRef]

18.   Chapman, D.P.; Presley-Cantrell, L.R.; Liu, Y.; Perry, G.S.; Wheaton, A.G.; Croft, J.B. Frequent insufficient sleep and anxiety and depressive disorders among US community dwellers in 20 states, 2010. *Psychiatr. Serv.* **2013**, *64*, 385–387. [CrossRef] [PubMed]

19.   Liu, Y.; Croft, J.B.; Wheaton, A.G.; Perry, G.S.; Chapman, D.P.; Strine, T.W.; McKnight-Eily, L.R.; Presley-Cantrell, L. Association between perceived insufficient sleep, frequent mental distress, obesity and chronic diseases among US adults, 2009 Behavioral Risk Factor Surveillance System. *BMC Public Health* **2013**, *13*, 84. [CrossRef]

20.   SAMHSA. 2014 National Survey on Drug Use and Health (NSDUH). Table 2.69B—Alcohol Use in the Past Month among Persons Aged 18 to 22, by College Enrollment Status and Demographic Characteristics: Percentages, 2013 and 2014. Available online: https://www.samhsa.gov/data/sites/default/files/NSDUH-DetTabs2014/NSDUH-DetTabs2014.pdf (accessed on 1 November 2018).

21.   Wheaton, A.G.; Olsen, E.O.; Miller, G.F.; Croft, J.B. Sleep Duration and Injury-Related Risk Behaviors Among High School Students—United States, 2007–2013. *Morb. Mortal. Wkly. Rep.* **2016**, *65*, 337–341. [CrossRef]

22.   Wong, M.M.; Roberson, G.; Dyson, R. Prospective relationship between poor sleep and substance-related problems in a national sample of adolescents. *Alcohol. Clin. Exp. Res.* **2015**, *39*, 355–362. [CrossRef]

23.   Short, M.A.; Louca, M. Sleep deprivation leads to mood deficits in healthy adolescents. *Sleep Med.* **2015**, *16*, 987–993. [CrossRef]

24.   Casement, M.D.; Keenan, K.E.; Hipwell, A.E.; Guyer, A.E.; Forbes, E.E. Neural reward processing mediates the relationship between insomnia symptoms and depression in adolescence. *Sleep* **2016**, *39*, 439–447. [CrossRef] [PubMed]

25.   Yoo, S.S.; Gujar, N.; Hu, P.; Jolesz, F.A.; Walker, M.P. The human emotional brain without sleep—a prefrontal amygdala disconnect. *Curr. Biol.* **2007**, *17*, R877–R878. [CrossRef] [PubMed]

26.   Berridge, K.C.; Robinson, T.E. Parsing reward. *Trends Neurosci.* **2003**, *26*, 507–513. [CrossRef]

27. Schultz, W. Behavioral theories and the neurophysiology of reward. *Annu. Rev. Psychol.* **2006**, *57*, 87–115. [CrossRef] [PubMed]

28. Knutson, B.; Wimmer, G.E. Splitting the difference: How does the brain code reward episodes? *Ann. N. Y. Acad. Sci.* **2007**, *1104*, 54–69. [CrossRef] [PubMed]

29. Boileau, I.; Assaad, J.M.; Pihl, R.O.; Benkelfat, C.; Leyton, M.; Diksic, M.; Tremblay, R.E.; Dagher, A. Alcohol promotes dopamine release in the human nucleus accumbens. *Synapse* **2003**, *49*, 226–231. [CrossRef]

30. Berridge, K.C.; Kringelbach, M.L. Affective neuroscience of pleasure: Reward in humans and animals. *Psychopharmacology* **2008**, *199*, 457–480. [CrossRef]

31. Grandner, M. Mind, body, and sport: Sleeping disorders. 2014. Available online: http://www.ncaa.org/health-and-safety/sport-science-institute/mind-body-and-sport-sleepingdisorders (accessed on 1 November 2018).

32. Leeder, J.; Glaister, M.; Pizzoferro, K.; Dawson, J.; Pedlar, C. Sleep duration and quality in elite athletes measured using wristwatch actigraphy. *J. Sports Sci.* **2012**, *30*, 541–545. [CrossRef]

33. Sexton-Radek, K.; Hernandez, A.; Pauley, S. Sleep quality in university/college athletes. *J. Sleep Disord. Ther.* **2013**, *2*, 144. [CrossRef]

34. American University/college Health Association. *ACHA-NCHA II Reference Group Data Report*; Reference Group Data Report—Spring 2015: Hanover, MD, USA, August 2015.

35. American Psychiatric Association. *Diagnostic and Statistical Manual of Mental Disorders*, 5th ed.; American Psychiatric Publishing: Arlington, VA, USA, 2013.

36. Altman, N.G.; Izci-Balserak, B.; Schopfer, E.; Jackson, N.; Rattanaumpawan, P.; Gehrman, P.R.; Patel, N.P.; Grandner, M.A. Sleep duration versus sleep insufficiency as predictors of cardiometabolic health outcomes. *Sleep Med.* **2012**, *13*, 1261–1270. [CrossRef]

37. Maia, Q.; Grandner, M.A.; Findley, J. Gurubhagavatula, I. Short and long sleep duration and risk of drowsy driving and the role of subjective sleep insufficiency. *Accid. Anal. Prev.* **2013**, *59*, 618–622. [CrossRef] [PubMed]

38. Grandner, M.A.; Jackson, N.J.; Izci-Balserak, B.; Gallagher, R.A.; Murray-Bachmann, R.; Williams, N.J.; Patel, N.P.; Jean-Louis, G. Social and behavioral determinants of perceived insufficient sleep. *Front. Neurol.* **2015**, *6*, 112. [CrossRef] [PubMed]

39. Presley, C.A.; Meilman, P.W.; Leichliter, J.S. University/college factors that influence drinking. *J. Stud. Alcohol Drugs* **2002**, *14*, 82–90.

40. Kenney, S.R.; LaBrie, J.W.; Hummer, J.F.; Pham, A.T. Global sleep quality as a moderator of alcohol consumption and consequences in university/college students. *Addict. Behav.* **2012**, *37*, 507–512. [CrossRef] [PubMed]

41. Kenney, S.R.; Paves, A.P.; Grimaldi, E.M.; LaBrie, J.W. Sleep quality and alcohol risk in university/college students: examining the moderating effects of drinking motives. *J. Am. Coll. Health* **2014**, *62*, 301–308. [CrossRef] [PubMed]

42. Baglioni, C.; Spiegelhalder, K.; Lombardo, C.; Riemann, D. Sleep and emotions: A focus on insomnia. *Sleep Med. Rev.* **2010**, *14*, 227–238. [CrossRef]

43. Curcio, G.; Ferrara, M.; De Gennaro, L. Sleep loss, learning capacity and academic performance. *Sleep Med. Rev.* **2006**, *10*, 323–337. [CrossRef]

44. Yusko, D.A.; Buckman, J.F.; White, H.R.; Pandina, R.J. Alcohol, tobacco, illicit drugs, and performance enhancers: A comparison of use by university/college student athletes and nonathletes. *J. Am. Coll. Health* **2008**, *57*, 281–290. [CrossRef]

45. Goudriaan, A.E.; Grekin, E.R.; Sher, K.J. Decision Making and Binge Drinking: A Longitudinal Study. *Alcohol. Clin. Exp. Res.* **2007**, *31*, 928–938. [CrossRef]

46. Dahl, R.; Gunnar, M. Heightened stress responsiveness and emotional reactivity during pubertal maturation: Implications for psychopathology. *Dev. Psychopathol.* **2009**, *21*, 1–6. [CrossRef]

47. Josephs, R.A.; Sellers, J.G.; Newman, M.L.; Mehta, P.H. The mismatch effect: When testosterone and status are at odds. *J. Personal. Soc. Psychol.* **2006**, *90*, 99–1013. [CrossRef] [PubMed]

48. Mazur, A.; Booth, A. Testosterone and dominance in men. *Behav. Brain Sci.* **1998**, *21*, 353–397. [CrossRef] [PubMed]

49. Steinberg, L. Risk taking in adolescence: What changes, and why? *Ann. N. Y. Acad. Sci.* **2004**, *1021*, 51–58. [CrossRef] [PubMed]

50. Turrisi, R.; Mastroleo, N.R.; Mallett, K.A.; Larimer, M.E.; Kilmer, J.R. Examination of the mediational influences of peer norms, environmental influences, and parent communications on heavy drinking in athletes and nonathletes. *Psychol. Addict. Behav.* **2007**, *21*, 453–461. [CrossRef] [PubMed]
51. Perkins, W. Surveying the damage: A review of research on consequences of alcohol misuse in university/college populations. *J. Stud. Alcohol Drugs* **2002**, *14*, 91–100. [CrossRef]
52. Prentice, D.A.; Miller, D.T. Pluralistic ignorance and alcohol use on campus: some consequences of misperceiving the social norm. *J. Personal. Soc. Psychol.* **1993**, *64*, 243–256. [CrossRef]
53. Galambos, N.L.; Dalton, A.L.; Maggs, J.L. Losing sleep over it: Daily variation in sleep quantity and quality in Canadian students' first semester of university/college. *J. Res. Adolesc.* **2009**, *19*, 741–761. [CrossRef]
54. Digdon, N.; Landry, K. University/college students' motives for drinking alcohol are related to evening preference, poor sleep, and ways of coping with stress. *Biol. Rhythm Res.* **2013**, *44*, 1–11. [CrossRef]

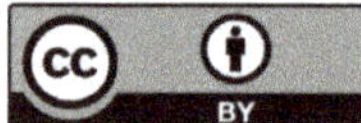

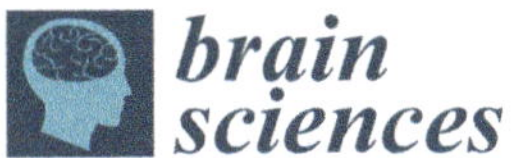 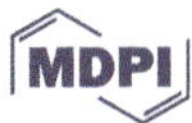

Review

Update on Insomnia after Mild Traumatic Brain Injury

Yi Zhou [1] and Brian D. Greenwald [2,*]

[1] Rutgers Robert Wood Johnson Medical School, Piscataway, NJ 08854, USA; yz411@scarletmail.rutgers.edu
[2] JFK Johnson Rehabilitation Institute, Edison, NJ 08820, USA
*   Correspondence: brian.greenwald@hackensackmeridian.org

Received: 18 November 2018; Accepted: 11 December 2018; Published: 13 December 2018

Abstract: Sleep disturbance after traumatic brain injury (TBI) has received growing interest in recent years, garnering many publications. Insomnia is highly prevalent within the mild traumatic brain injury (mTBI) population and is a subtle, frequently persistent complaint that often goes undiagnosed. For individuals with mTBI, problems with sleep can compromise the recovery process and impede social reintegration. This article updates the evidence on etiology, epidemiology, prognosis, consequences, differential diagnosis, and treatment of insomnia in the context of mild TBI. This article aims to increase awareness about insomnia following mTBI in the hopes that it may improve diagnosis, evaluation, and treatment of sleeping disturbance in this population while revealing areas for future research.

Keywords: mild traumatic brain injury; mTBI; concussion; insomnia; sleep disturbance; treatment

---

1. Methods

References for this narrative review were obtained using a search of online databases PUBMED, MEDLINE, CINAL, and COCHRANE (Figure 1). These online databases were used to search for papers published after the year 2000 using keywords: mild traumatic brain injury, mTBI, concussion, insomnia, sleep disturbance, and treatment. Boolean operator "AND" was used to connect search terms and narrow results. Truncations and MeSH headings were not used. Some references were not identified using the online databases, but were obtained through reference lists of other articles. Our inclusion criteria were studies that looked primarily at brain injury cases, specifically mild traumatic brain injury. Only papers printed in or translated into English were included. We excluded case reports as sources.

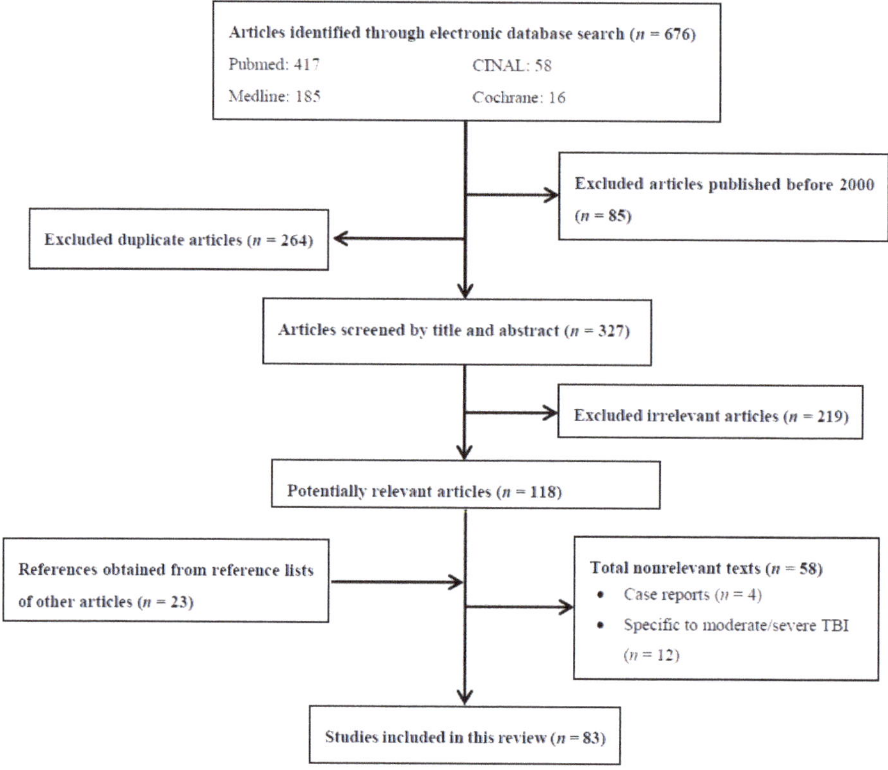

Figure 1. Process flow chart.

2. Introduction

Traumatic brain injury (TBI) is a leading cause of disability in the United States. The Center for Disease Control and Prevention recently reported that in 2013 there were 2.8 million cases of TBI-related ER visits, hospitalizations, and deaths [1]. Of the annual cases of traumatic brain injury, the World Health Organization estimates that 70% to 90% of those are mild TBI [2]. The most common groups to sustain a mild TBI are males, teenagers, and young adults, while the most common causes are falls, motor-vehicle collisions, and assault [2]. Despite the high incidence, mTBI numbers are likely an underestimation [1]. One study found that in the emergency department, 56% of cases that qualified as mTBI did not carry a documented diagnosis, suggesting that many patients are potentially undiagnosed [3]. One proposed reason mTBI is frequently missed is that standard imaging in patients with mTBI does not show hemorrhage or other obvious structural abnormalities [4]. Likewise, mTBI-associated sleep disturbances are often unnoticed in the ED and primary care clinics as providers tend to focus on vision changes, nausea, vomiting, head and neck pain [5]. This suggests a need for a higher index of suspicion, targeted questioning and appropriate screening tools to improve diagnosis of both mTBI and associated sleep disturbance [6].

According to the American Congress of Rehabilitation Medicine (ACRM), mild traumatic brain injury is defined as traumatically induced physiologic disruption of brain function that manifests with at least one of the following: any period of loss of consciousness (LOC), memory loss before or after injury, alteration in mental state at time of injury (i.e., feeling dazed, disoriented, confused) or focal neurological deficit(s) that may or may not be transient [7]. Classification as mild requires that severity does not exceed a Glasgow Coma Scale (GCS) score between 13 and 15 after 30 min, a PTA of greater than 24 h, or LOC of more than 30 min [5]. Common symptoms associated with mTBI include headache, dizziness, bad taste, sleep disturbance, nausea/vomiting, impaired balance and coordination, tinnitus, and vision changes [8]. TBI also results in significant cognitive, emotional, and behavioral disorders which all increase morbidity [9]. Poor sleep may develop acutely and last several years post-injury and is described by those who experience a mild TBI as one of the most debilitating consequences [10].

3. Pathophysiology of Sleep Disturbance after TBI

Traumatic brain injury is classified into primary and secondary brain injury. Primary injury refers to the structural damage created upon impact. Secondary injury refers to the damage from subsequent cellular processes following primary injury such as excitotoxicity, free radical generation, calcium-mediated damage, hypoxia, and increased intracranial pressure [11,12]. Unsurprisingly, these mechanisms can incur structural, biochemical, and genetic changes implicated in sleep disturbance.

Coup–countrecoup injury typically occurs at the base of the skull in areas of bony prominences so the anterior temporal and inferior frontal regions, including the basal forebrain, are frequently injured. Since the basal forebrain contributes to sleep initiation, injury to this region can lead to insomnia symptoms [8]. The structure of the tentorium has also been associated with sleep pathology. When controlling for cognitive function and mTBI severity, researchers found those with sleep–wake disturbances had longer tentorial lengths and flatter angles, suggesting closer proximity of the tentorial edge to the pineal gland. The authors reason this proximity increases the risk of direct impact between the tentorium and pineal gland subsequently disrupting melatonin pathways [13]. Another study with mTBI patients measured fractional anisotropy (FA) with MRI as a representation of white matter integrity. In patients with sleep disturbance there was reduced parahippocampal FA, which was strikingly similar to findings of early Alzheimer dementia, in which sleep–wake disturbance is one of the earliest symptoms [14]. Using rodent models of TBI, researchers found increased reactive microglia in the thalamus preceding development of sleep disruption. The authors postulate that the inflammatory response may interfere with the thalamocortical network, which regulates sleep–wake patterns [15].

Sleep disturbance after TBI is associated with numerous biochemical changes as well. One study demonstrated lower evening melatonin production in TBI patients compared to healthy controls, which was associated with decreased sleep efficiency, increased wake after sleep onset (WASO), and higher rates of depression and anxiety [16]. Decreased melatonin likely arises from the aforementioned pathway disruptions and/or damage to the suprachiasmatic nucleus [8]. Other reported biochemical associations include changes in levels of hypocretin-1, dopamine, and serotonin, which are neurotransmitters involved in sleep modulation [17]. Decreased levels of IGF-I and testosterone were also found specifically after blast-induced mTBI [18]. More on the distinction of mTBI from blast injury is discussed in Section 5.1.

A variety of genes involved in inflammation, glial function, neuronal plasticity, immunity, and circadian rhythm have implications on sleep disturbance post-TBI [19]. For example, in rodent models several plasticity genes like *Bdnf*, *Homer1a*, and *Fos* have decreased expression a few days after mTBI. This is important because these plasticity genes have demonstrated roles in maintaining sleep homeostasis [19]. Also, in rodent models the astrocyte marker *Gfap* was elevated in the cortex after TBI and prior to the development of sleep disruptions, suggesting that astrocyte activation may contribute to sleep modification [15,19]. In mTBI patients, one of the clock genes, *PERIOD3* (*PER3*), was found to be associated with changes in sleep recovery. Specifically, the *PER3* gene carries a polymorphism that comes in either 4 or 5 tandem repeats and patients who were carriers of 5 repeats interestingly reported improved sleep quality but shorter sleep duration compared to noncarriers at 6 weeks post-mTBI [20].

Sleep Architecture Changes Seen after mTBI

Sleep architecture refers to the organization and cyclical pattern of normal sleep with specific corresponding electroencephalographic (EEG) activities [21]. Sleep is comprised of slow-wave sleep and paradoxical sleep. Within slow-wave sleep there are 4 stages. Stages 1 and 2 are considered light sleep, while stages 3 and 4 are considered deep sleep. These stages can fall under the term "non-rapid eye movement (NREM) sleep". The paradoxical sleep stage involves rapid eye movement (REM) sleep which has similar EEG activity to wakefulness and is the stage in which dreaming occurs [21]. In adults, NREM takes up about 20% of the night, while REM takes up about 80% and each stage of sleep is thought to perform independent yet complementary restorative functions [4].

When it comes to sleep architecture after mild TBI, patients generally experience "sleep fragmentation" referring to reduced total sleep time and a greater proportion of sleep in light sleep stages [20]. Observed changes of sleep in mTBI patients include increased stages 1 and 2 sleep and decreased REM sleep [17,22,23]. One study also found no significant difference in sleep and REM latencies in mTBI patients compared to controls [22].

Even though absence of objective findings is common in mTBI patients reporting sleep disturbance, studies recommend that the subjective experience should take precedence [17,22,24]. While mTBI patients with insomnia also tend to underestimate the time spent asleep, subjective sleep is still predictive of depression, anxiety, and general distress [25,26]. As insomnia is by definition a subjective complaint, it is important not to disregard patients even in the absence of objective evidence.

4. Insomnia and mTBI

Insomnia is characterized by poor sleep quantity or quality in the forms of delayed sleep onset, nocturnal awakenings with difficulty returning to sleep, waking too early, and not feeling rested despite adequate sleep hours. A required criterion for diagnosing insomnia of any form is that it leads to distress and subjective impairment in the daytime [27]. Insomnia is important to address as it affects patients both psychologically and cognitively throughout recovery and impedes a patient's return to normal functioning.

Sleep disorders such as insomnia, sleep apnea, narcolepsy, periodic limb movement disorder are all more prevalent in TBI patients compared to the general population [28]. Insomnia is the most commonly reported sleep disturbance with approximately 40%–65% of mTBI patients reporting symptoms of insomnia [12]. However, there are conflicting findings on whether insomnia among TBI patients are over- or underreported. In a survey of 452 patients with TBI, the majority of which were severe TBI (59.9%), 50.2% reported insomnia symptoms, while only 29.4% fulfilled the DSM-IV diagnosis of insomnia [29]. Another study of mTBI patients by Sullivan et al. found that although 42% of their sample had insomnia, only 16% self-reported an insomnia diagnosis [30]. The contrary findings may suggest an association between severity of brain injury and insomnia symptoms, a relationship that will be further discussed in Section 5.2.

A popular model of insomnia contains two components, a general predisposition to developing insomnia followed by an acute stressor [17]. There are various interpretations on how this model applies to TBI. In one interpretation, those suffering from insomnia post-TBI may have had previous episodes of insomnia or a family history. The acute stressor would therefore be the TBI itself [17]. Another interpretation surmises that both aspects of the model may be affected by TBI because pathophysiological changes of the brain create a predisposition for insomnia while acute stressors come in the forms of comorbidities such as pain, depression, and anxiety [11,18]. TBI patients will also often experience multiple psychosocial stressors simultaneously such as inability to return to work, financial difficulties, redefined familial roles, and strained social relationships. Increased familial discord, marital problems, and litigation procedures have been documented with TBI patients and are obvious sources of significant stress [31]. The patient experience and environment are therefore important to consider in management of these patients.

5. Epidemiology of Insomnia after mTBI

Within the general population, sufferers of insomnia are more likely to be white, older, female, and unmarried. Although prevalence of insomnia symptoms increases with age in the general population, sleep dissatisfaction and diagnoses were found to be independent of age [32]. The demographic characteristics differ in the context of TBI as a study by Fichtenberg et al. of patients with various severities of TBI found no relationship between insomnia and gender, age, or education [33]. In the mTBI population, age at time of injury may have implications on the development of insomnia. For example, adolescence is a time of increased risk for sleep problems due to physiologic changes and increased societal and academic demands. Thus, when adolescents experience a mild TBI they have a higher predispositon than younger children to develop chronic sleep problems [34]. It is generally believed that TBI outcomes like sleep disturbance worsen with increased age possibly due to reasons such as decreased ability to compensate, decreased cerebral reserve, and pre-existing comorbidities [35]. When it comes to mTBI, literature remains divided on how age affects outcomes [35]. Some studies suggest increased symptom severity with age; however, a study by Hu et al. found that middle-aged mTBI patients (36–55 years) had a higher severity of sleep disturbance compared to elderly patients [35]. The authors suggest that this finding may be due to middle-aged patients noticing more significant deviations from their baseline functional status and experiencing more daily stressors such as employment and living with dependents. Although studies are revealing potential risk factors, further research is needed to better comprehend the risk factors that predispose and precipitate insomnia after mild TBI.

5.1. Repeat TBI and Blast Injury

Repeat mTBIs are found to increase the likelihood and severity of insomnia as well as cause persistent deficits in spatial learning and memory, subacute anxiety, and depression relative to the aftermath of a single mTBI [36]. A study of military personnel found that 20% of patients with a single mTBI reported insomnia, whereas 50% of patients who experienced multiple mTBIs reported insomnia [37]. It is worth noting that blast injury accounts for around 60% of military-related TBIs of which 80% are classified as mild TBI [38]. Unlike blunt trauma associated with other forms of TBI, blast injury produces shockwaves that create propagating pressure transients that can lead to diffuse axonal injury, contusion, edema, and hemorrhage [39]. This describes only primary blast injury and it is also important to consider potential damage from shrapnel, thermal effects of detonation, and psychological consequences [39]. In a broad context, TBI and blast-related TBI (bTBI) are often discussed in the same vein because evidence points to similar impairments after injury. One study comparing bTBI to other causes of brain injury found no significant differences in sleep impairment along with cognitive impairment, pain, and other symptoms post-injury [40]. However, distinct consequences of bTBI include hearing loss, tinnitus, and increased incidence of post-traumatic stress disorder (PTSD) symptoms [39]. Therefore, consequences of blast-related TBI compared to those from other forms of TBI are not synonymous and differences are important to keep in mind in practice and literature. Regarding repeat TBIs, sleep disturbance is itself a risk factor for repeat brain injury. Insomnia is known to increase the risk of industrial and vehicle accidents, thereby increasing risk of TBI and reoccurrence [27]. One survey found that chronic insomnia doubled the risk of automobile accidents due to sleepiness [41]. Since insomnia after TBI increases risk for reoccurrence, safety precautions and follow-up should be emphasized.

5.2. Implications of TBI Severity

A frequently mentioned and somewhat counterintuitive finding is that mild TBI is more strongly associated with insomnia and other sleep disturbances compared to more severe TBI [35]. Opposition to this correlation includes a prospective study by Baumann et al., which found that severity of inciting head injury did not predict sleep–wake disturbances [42]. Despite this finding, evidence generally supports the relationship between insomnia and milder TBI [29,33,43]. The higher prevalence of insomnia in mTBI patients may be secondary to increased awareness of impairment and disability leading to an increase in self-reporting [33]. Mild TBI patients may also be under more pressure to reintegrate into normal life which could lead to increased stress and sleep issues [8,35].

6. Prognosis

Prognosis of mTBI is typically good with one study finding that almost all previously healthy adults (96%) return to work/normal activities within one year post-mTBI [44]. Despite this prognosis, a large prospective cohort study discovered a that significant minority of patients after mild TBI, around 20%, are not functionally recovered even by one year post-injury [45]. Sleep difficulty is one of the postconcussive symptoms that is assumed to resolve spontaneously over time. Along with depression and anxiety, all are expected to improve; however, one study found that only sleep quality improved to the pre-mTBI level by 6 weeks [46]. This implies that recovery from sleep disturbance is relatively rapid, yet studies that extend beyond the subacute stage suggest otherwise. For example, a study found that for veterans with mTBI, poor sleep quality lasted on average 6 years post-injury and was independent of combat exposure, PTSD, mood disorders, anxiety, and substance use [47].

It is generally accepted that negative outcomes of mTBI resolve even more rapidly within the younger population with complete recovery expected within 2–3 months for children and adolescents [34]. However, a longitudinal study of children between the ages of 8–16 years found little improvement in sleep difficulties after 6 months and 28% still experienced poor sleep at one year post-mTBI [48]. In the study, sleep quality at 1 month was predictive of symptom severity and behavioral outcomes at 12 months, suggesting that prompt intervention may facilitate recovery [48]. Persistent sleep impairment among the younger population is reinforced with another study that found that around a third of adolescents after mTBI had greater levels of sleep disturbance compared to healthy peers even 6 years after injury [49]. These findings appear to counter the common belief of mTBI's speedy recovery especially in younger patients. While other symptoms post-mTBI may resolve, these study findings (further detailed in Table 1) suggest that sleep disturbance persists for years in a significant proportion of patients regardless of age group.

Table 1. Summary of study findings of sleep disturbance chronicity after mild traumatic brain injury (mTBI).

Study	Study Design	Participants	Sleep Outcome Measure	Results	Limitations
Ma et al. (2014) [46]	Prospective cohort	mTBI group: · $n = 100$ · Age: >20 years, (mean = 38.88 years) Control group: · $n = 137$, · Age: >20 years (mean: 29.86 years) · without TBI	Pittsburgh Sleep Quality Index (PSQI)	· Baseline mTBI PSQI scores significantly different from scores of control · At 6 weeks follow-up, mTBI PSQI scores improved significantly and were not significantly different from scores of control	· Medication use may have interfered with assessment · Unidentified pre-existing comorbidities · Only evaluated subacute stage of sleep quality · Self-report
McMahon et al. (2014) [45]	Prospective cohort	mTBI study population: · $n = 375$ · Age: >18 years, (mean = 44 years)	Postconcussion Syndrome (PCS) Symptom Checklist	· At 3 months, 50.2% of mTBI patients report at least one sleep symptom ($n = 348$) · At 1 year follow-up, 53.5% of mTBI patients report at least one sleep symptom ($n = 199$)	· No control group · Loss of patients to follow-up · Did not analyze contribution of medical history on outcome · Self-report
Martindale et al. (2017) [47]	Cross-sectional	mTBI study population: · Veterans ($n = 527$) · Age: >21 years, (mean = 35.47 years)	Pittsburgh Sleep Quality Index (PSQI)	· 56.2% of sample reported clinically significant poor sleep quality · Poor sleep quality lasts on average 6 years independent of combat exposure, post-traumatic stress disorder (PTSD), mood disorders, anxiety disorders, and substance use disorders	· Deployment related-mTBI limits generalizability · Cross-sectional data, unable to evaluate temporal relationship · Self-report
Theadom and Parag et al. (2016) [50]	Longitudinal population study	mTBI study population: · $n = 341$ · Age: >16 years, (mean = 37.5 years)	Rivermead Post Concussion Symptoms Questionnaire (RPQ)	· 43% of sample reported sleep disturbance at baseline · At 12 months 32% still reported sleep disturbance	· Lack of information on prior mood, psychiatric and medical conditions · Self-report

Table 1. *Cont.*

Study	Study Design	Participants	Sleep Outcome Measure	Results	Limitations
Theadom and Starkey et al. (2016) [48]	Prospective cohort	mTBI group: · $n = 109$ · Age: 8–16 years, (mean = 11.49 years) Control group: · $n = 68$, · Age: 8–16 years (mean: 11.52 years) · Without TBI	Pittsburgh Sleep Quality Index (PSQI)	· At 12 months, 28% of mTBI group reported poor sleep quality compared to 39% at 1 month · mTBI group had significantly poorer sleep quality compared to healthy controls (OR = 3.09) at 12 months post-injury	· Data from parent reporting
Pillar et al. (2003) [49]	Cross-sectional	mTBI group: · $n = 98$ · Age: 8–18 years, (mean = 13.5 years) · 0.5–6 years post-injury at time of study Control group: · $n = 80$, · Age: 8–18 years (mean: 12.4 years) · Without TBI	Study designed questionnaire	· 28% of mTBI group reported long-term sleep disturbance (6 months to 6 years) compared to 11% of controls	· Did not stratify findings based on mTBI chronicity · Cross-sectional data, unable to evaluate temporal relationship · Self-report · Response rate (98/150) may inflate prevalence

Consequences of Sleep Impairment

Sleep quality impacts all areas of daily functioning and is also crucial for the recovery process. Memory, attention, and executive functions are the cognitive domains most affected by sleep impairment [51]. This aligns with recent evidence demonstrating the importance of sleep on neural growth and plasticity, learning, and memory consolidation [4]. Poor sleep was found to be significantly predictive of poorer post-concussion symptoms, mood, community integration, and cognitive ability at one year post-injury [52]. Sleep disruption may also act as a cellular stressor and lead to cognitive decline. Studies found that disrupted sleep leads to accumulation of hyperphosphorylated tau and amyloid beta plaque accumulation from oxidative stress [23].

Fatigue is a common sequelae post-mTBI that emerges as soon as a few days post-injury [53]. There exist two supported models of cognitive fatigue after mTBI, including fatigue secondary to increased work to process information and fatigue secondary to impaired sleep [54]. One study found the prevalence of fatigue to be 68% at one week post-mTBI and decrease to 38% after 3 months [55]. Although fatigue is found to be higher at the 4 month mark in mTBI compared to sTBI, fatigue tends to reduce over time after mild TBI and increase after severe [53]. However, even by 6 months after sustaining an mTBI, 32%–34% of individuals reported fatigue [55,56]. The concern regarding the high prevalence of fatigue in the mTBI population is association with higher reported levels of functional impairment, depression, and cognitive difficulties [53,56].

For adolescents, studies find that persistent sleep impairment following mTBI is associated with poorer quality of life, greater depressive symptoms and decreased participation in normal roles [34]. In a study of university students (18–25 years) with mTBI, sleep impairment led to increased daytime dysfunction along with lower levels of enthusiasm and energy in completing tasks. Participants also experienced behavioral problems which were moderately correlated with sleep-related daytime dysfunction in the forms of social withdrawal, poor relationships, clumsiness, and speech difficulties [57]. The consequences of poor sleep in these populations are particularly detrimental during a time when social integration, academic functioning, and development are critical.

Within the working population, individuals with sleep impairment present with greater absenteeism, increased presenteeism, lower job satisfaction and work productivity loss [27,41]. In a study of workers with delayed recovery from mTBI, insomnia was the only variable associated with greater odds of disability while age, sex, education, income, and marital status were not associated with greater perceived disability [58]. Therefore, prioritizing sleep management in these patients may expedite return to normal functioning and mitigate potential sources of stress.

7. Differential Diagnosis of Sleep Disturbance after TBI

7.1. Pain

Pain is one of the most frequent complaints post-mTBI and along with insufficient management is a significant contributor to sleep disturbance [59]. Comorbid pain was found in over 60% of mTBI patients and often presented in the forms of headaches, joint, neck, shoulder and back pain [59–61]. Similar to the trends of sleep disturbance, reports of pain are more frequent in the mTBI population than in more severe injuries. A possible explanation is that patients with severe injuries are often bedridden and treated with paralytic agents allowing healing of cervical injuries. Those with mild injuries may continue to use those damaged muscles and ligaments, thereby interfering with healing [62]. Those with severe injuries may also have more difficulty communicating their pain to providers [62]. In early recovery, Suzuki et al. observed that pain increased sleep need to over 8 h in a third of mTBI patients [60]. In mTBI patients with pain, fast beta and gamma electroencephalographic activity were observed in frontal, central, and occipital electroencephalographic (EEG) within all sleep stages. This finding suggests that the increased need for sleep is secondary to persistent wake EEG activity, leading to unrestful sleep [59]. Evaluation of pain is a necessary precursor to the management of new sleep complaints after mTBI as adequate pain management may treat insomnia as well.

7.2. Sleep Apnea

Behind insomnia, sleep apnea is one of the most frequently diagnosed sleep disorders post-TBI [28]. Both obstructive and central sleep apneas are more prevalent in the TBI population and seem to arise from a complex interaction between brain injury, decreased arousal, and impaired respiratory effort [6,63]. Obstructive sleep apnea (OSA) refers to intermittent episodes of upper airway obstruction that reduces blood oxygenation [28]. Studies have demonstrated prevalence of obstructive sleep apnea to be 25% to 35% following TBI of any severity which is substantially higher than general population findings [63].

While many patients complain of insomnia and will lack objective findings, patients with diagnosable sleep apnea will often fail to recognize the problem and only describe poor day time vigilance [28]. Although costly and time-consuming, the gold standard for diagnosing sleep apnea is polysomnography (PSG), which will commonly find increased sleep onset latency, poor sleep efficiency, and decreased REM latency [6]. Sleep apnea is predictive of higher all-cause mortality and recurrent vascular events after stroke and TIA implying urgency in diagnosing and treating sleep-disordered breathing within the TBI population [6]. It is worth noting that studies that found sleep apnea of any severity significantly increases risk of TBI [64]. Therefore, sleep apnea may also be an important target in the prevention of TBI. Treatment is unchanged to those with other causes of sleep-disordered breathing where positive airway pressure (PAP) is the standard of care [4].

7.3. Post-Traumatic Stress Disorder

The majority of studies on the relationship between post-traumatic stress disorder (PTSD) and traumatic brain injury understandably involve veterans where the rate of PTSD after TBI ranges from around 27% to 44% [65]. Among the civilian population suffering from nonmilitary trauma, one study found that 14% to 56% of TBI patients had comorbid PTSD [65]. PTSD is diagnosed via criteria released by the American Psychiatric Association which shares many symptoms with TBI, often causing attribution of symptoms to be difficult [66]. One of the shared and core symptoms of PTSD is sleep disturbance, found in around 70% of PTSD patients [12]. Although it is difficult in PTSD–TBI comorbid patients to assess the roles each play in sleep impairment, certain sleep pathology may be distinguishable between the two. One study comparing TBI and PTSD patients among returning veterans found no differences in the rates of OSA, excessive awakenings and daytime sleepiness but on PSG, PTSD patients demonstrated greater arousal frequency while TBI patients demonstrated greater slow-wave sleep [67].

Similar to symptoms, the treatment of sleep disturbance in PTSD and TBI patients overlaps. Despite similarities, certain treatments may be prioritized depending on the presence of comorbid PTSD with TBI. VA/DOD Clinical Practice Guidelines for the treatment of PTSD recommend prazosin, an alpha-1 adrenergic antagonist, as treatment for sleep impairment and nightmares in PTSD [65,66]. Other supported pharmacologic options for PTSD include venlafaxine, a serotonin norepinephrine reuptake inhibitor (SNRI), and selective serotonin inhibitors such as sertraline and paroxetine [65]. Likewise, cognitive behavioral therapy (CBT) is a mainstay of treatment for sleep impairment in TBI but studies recommend trauma-focused CBT for comorbid PTSD in reducing symptoms [65]. For these patients, there is likely a complex interplay between TBI and PTSD that results in sleep impairment and currently cannot be separated into exclusive contributions. Therefore, more research is needed in studying the associations between sleep disturbance and TBI patients with comorbid PTSD. Recommended management of sleep disturbance in the PTSD population differs slightly from TBI and is therefore up to clinical judgment for attempting PTSD targeted treatments.

7.4. Circadian Rhythm

Circadian rhythm disorders are sometimes mistaken for insomnia post-TBI. Circadian rhythm disorder refers to disruption of the normal 24 hr cycle of body patterns such as body temperature and melatonin secretion [10,23]. Circadian sleep disturbances come in the forms of irregular sleep–wake pattern and more commonly delayed sleep phase syndrome [68]. A study by Ayalon et al., using actigraphy, salivary melatonin, temperature measurement, and polysomnography, found that 36% of patients who were diagnosed with insomnia actually had circadian sleep disturbance [68]. The distinction between insomnia and circadian rhythm disorder is important as treatment differs. Rather than prescribe hypnotics, melatonin or bright light therapy are more appropriate for these patients [68].

8. Treatment

Many treatment options are available for patients suffering from insomnia post-TBI (Table 2). Despite this, insomnia is often undertreated and patients seek treatment independent of health care providers in the forms of over-the-counter (OTC) medications and alcohol [69]. In the context of TBI, one study found that around 60% of those fulfilling diagnosis of insomnia were left untreated [29].

Similar to the management of most chronic medical conditions, providers should begin with conservative measures and proceed to more aggressive options only when necessary. As was discussed, this begins with ruling out common comorbidities as causes of sleep impairment. After other etiologies are considered, further interventions can be sought.

8.1. Sleep Hygiene

Sleep hygiene is a broad term that refers to adjustments that improve sleep health. The basis is to replace stimulating behaviors with sleep-promoting behaviors. Examples of adjustments include exercising, consuming a snack before bed, keeping the bedroom dark, limiting noise, maintaining a regular sleep schedule, and reducing intake of stimulants and alcohol [70]. Individuals with chronic insomnia will often spend more time in bed and nap during the day leading to irregular sleep–wake schedules. These behaviors likely desynchronize the natural cycle and contribute to sleep disturbances [31]. Many studies advocate sleep hygiene incorporation into the care plans of TBI patients as it is low cost, low risk, and noninvasive [71]. Studies have demonstrated that increased knowledge of sleep hygiene post-TBI was associated with better sleep habits and subsequent sleep quality improvements [72].

8.2. Cognitive Behavioral Therapy & Digital CBT

Cognitive behavioral therapy (CBT) encompasses sleep hygiene along with other techniques such as relaxation, sleep restriction, and stimulus control. The goal of CBT is to reduce unrealistic expectations and anxiety towards sleep by identifying and mitigating deleterious thoughts surrounding and during sleep [70]. A key component of CBT is the sleep diary that includes self–reported data on time in bed, medication use, caffeine intake, exercise, and awakenings as an attempt to eliminate recall bias [70]. A systematic review by Bogdanov et al. demonstrated significant improvements in insomnia severity and sleep diary data after CBT among patients with TBI and comorbid insomnia. The benefits of CBT were found to appear within 1–2 weeks of implementation and sustained by time of follow-up 3 months later [73]. Another study found that patients undergoing CBT also had significant improvements in both fatigue and depression that persisted at follow-up 2 months later [74]. These findings support why CBT is widely advocated as a standard of care for insomnia including within the TBI population.

Table 2. Pros/Cons of Commonly Used Treatments for Insomnia after TBI.

Intervention	Pros	Cons
Sleep Hygiene Counseling	· Effective in improving sleep quality and reducing daytime sleepiness · Inexpensive, low risk, noninvasive · Persistent improvement on sleep · Recommendations may be catered to patient environment	· Variable recommendations, provider-dependent · Issue of non-compliance · Patients may be non-receptive to indirect intervention · Barriers may exist for implementing changes (ex. living arrangement, occupation, economic status, disability, dependents, etc.)
Cognitive Behavioral Therapy (CBT)	· Effective in improving insomnia severity, sleep efficiency, and quality · Includes sleep hygiene counseling · Low risk, noninvasive · Benefits appear within 1–2 weeks · Persistent improvement on sleep · Persistent improvement in comorbid fatigue, depression and anxiety · Newer digital CBT may address accessibility and scalability	· Time commitment (meetings, maintaining sleep diary) · Issue of noncompliance · Financial costs · Provider dependent efficacy · Variable settings (one to one or in group settings)
Benzodiazepines (i.e., flurazepam, lorazepam, estazolam)	· Effective in increasing total sleep time and improving sleep quality	· Risk of dependency and abuse · Associated with daytime sedation and cognitive impairment · Increases risk of falls/accidents · Short-term benefit

Table 2. *Cont.*

Intervention	Pros	Cons
Z-drugs (i.e., zaleplon, zolpidem, zopiclone)	· Effective in increasing total sleep time and improving sleep quality · Well tolerated, no daytime cognitive or psychomotor impairment · Significantly lower incidence of dependence compared to benzodiazepines	· Associated with daytime sedation · Potential psychological dependency and abuse potential · May cause sensory distortions · Short term benefit · Lack of research in TBI patients
Trazodone	· Increases sleep duration in insomnia and with comorbid depression · Generally well tolerated · Comparable antidepressant effect to selective serotonin reuptake inhibitors (SSRI) and tricyclic antidepressants(TCA) · Decreased anticholinergic effects compared to TCA	· Associated with daytime sedation, headache, dry mouth, sexual dysfunction, orthostatic hypotension · Short-term benefit · Lack of research in TBI patients
Melatonin & Melatonin Agonists (i.e., ramelteon, tasimelteon)	· Increases total sleep time and decreases sleep latency · OTC melatonin affordable and accessible · No risk of dependency or tolerance	· Agonists are costly · Short-term benefit

Available pharmacologic and non-pharmacologic interventions for treatment of insomnia. [70–83].

"Digital CBT" has received growing interest in recent years and is a general term referring to CBT provided via web and mobile platforms [75]. A recent RCT comparing dCBT to sleep hygiene counseling for general insomnia found small improvements in functional health and psychological well-being, but large improvements in sleep-related quality of life and insomnia symptoms [76]. When comparing dCBT to CBT, meta-analyses demonstrate that the effects of dCBT on insomnia at increasing total sleep time, decreasing sleep onset latency and decreasing WASO are in the ranges of conventional CBT, suggesting similar effectiveness [75] Relative to CBT, dCBT also tended to be more cost-effective with lower societal and healthcare costs [75]. Besides similar efficacy and improved cost-effectiveness, dCBT's ability to disseminate effective treatment for insomnia is likely its greatest advantage [75]. Although dCBT appears to be a promising avenue for treatment, much research is needed on the effects of dCBT for insomnia post-TBI.

9. Pharmacologic Options

9.1. Benzodiazepines/Z-Drugs

Benzodiazepines such as diazepam, lorazepam, and alprazolam have largely fallen out of use due to side effects such as dependency, daytime sedation, cognitive impairment, and increased risk of falls/accidents that are deleterious to recovery from TBI [77]. The Z-drugs (zapleplon, zopiclone, and zolpidem) are alternatives. Similar to benzodiazepines, Z-drugs are also GABA agonists but act more specifically on the type 1 receptor [78]. Z-drugs are not without their potential side effects, including daytime sedation and sensory distortions, but generally have no daytime consequences on cognitive and psychomotor function. Z-drugs also have shorter half-lives compared to benzodiazepines ranging from 1 hr with zapleplon to 5 hrs with zopiclone. It is believed that the selective target and faster offset of action contribute to the preferable side effect profile of Z-drugs as compared to benzodiazepines [78]. While Z-drugs have a significantly lower incidence of dependence relative to benzodiazepines, there is still a risk of abuse especially in patients with a history of substance abuse, dependence, or psychiatric diseases [79]. Research on the efficacy of Z-drugs within the TBI population is limited. One study comparing the efficacies of lorazepam and zopiclone in treating insomnia for stroke and brain injury patients found that both groups slept more than 7 h and did not differ in quality of sleep, suggesting similar effectiveness [80]. Long-term therapeutic benefits of both benzodiazepines and Z-drugs are limited, so while indicated for short-term use, one should defer to attempting non-pharmacologic treatments.

9.2. Trazodone

Trazodone is a heterocyclic antidepressant and one of the most frequently prescribed drugs for treatment of insomnia in TBI patients [78]. Its mechanism in humans remains poorly understood; however, animal models have shown that trazodone inhibits serotonin re-uptake [78]. For TBI patients, trazodone is generally well tolerated and unlike the tricyclic antidepressants, has little to no anticholinergic effect [81]. Compared to Z-drugs, trazodone has a relatively longer half-life at 5–9 h, so daytime sedation is a potential side effect [81]. Despite trazodone's usage, there are no clinical trials on trazodone for insomnia treatment in the TBI population. For insomnia in the general population, trazodone increased sleep duration compared to placebo and in patients with comorbid depression was also found to increase total sleep time [78]. As depression is a common comorbidity in patients with TBI, trazodone may be first line for select patients.

9.3. Melatonin/Melatonin Agonists

Melatonin is a hormone synthesized in the pineal gland that is triggered by the absence of light and plays a crucial role in the sleep–wake cycle. As mentioned, TBI patients tend to have disruptions in the melatonin pathways, which result in lower melatonin levels later in the day compared to healthy controls [16]. A RCT comparing the efficacy of melatonin supplementation to placebo for TBI patients with sleep disturbance found improved sleep quality, sleep efficiency, and decreased anxiety with no significant difference in sleep latency [82].

Efficacy of exogenous melatonin has led to the development of melatonin agonist ramelteon. Similar to melatonin supplementation, ramelteon has a superior side effect profile [78]. In a pilot study investigating the effects of ramelteon on sleep among patients with TBI, patients were given 8 mg nightly over 3 weeks. The study demonstrated a significant increase in total sleep time and a modest improvement in sleep latency compared to placebo. On standardized neuropsychological testing, participants also had improved scores particularly in executive functioning [83]. Currently, no generic formulation is commercially available so as melatonin agonists increase in popularity, they may become more affordable and viable options.

10. Summary and Conclusions

Insomnia is a highly prevalent and debilitating condition within the mTBI population with around 40%–65% of patients reporting symptoms of insomnia. As both mTBI and associated insomnia are underdiagnosed, a proper history and high clinical suspicion are important in detecting underlying sleep disorder. Although most patients with mTBI return to normal functioning, sleep disturbance is a subtle and often persistent condition lasting many years for a significant proportion of patients. Since many brain injury patients self-treat and feel lost when addressing these new sleep disturbances, it is important for providers to follow up with patients regarding sleep post-TBI and maintain a low threshold to intervene as poor sleep hinders recovery and social reintegration. When addressing impaired sleep, rule out common comorbidities prior to management as treatment may differ. Pharmacologic options are effective for situational use but may have negative consequences in the long term. As sleep impairment may last years after injury, attempting nonpharmacologic treatments such as sleep hygiene counseling and CBT are preferred as they demonstrate persistent benefits. Since mild TBI is by far the most common severity of TBI and data suggests that milder brain injury increases risk of insomnia, more research is needed towards studying insomnia and its treatment within the mild traumatic brain injury population.

Funding: This research received no external funding.

Acknowledgments: We want to thank Rutgers Robert Wood Johnson Medical School and JFK Johnson Rehabilitation Institute for allowing us to do this work. We would also like to thank our peers and friends for providing support and advice along the way.

References

1. Taylor, C.A.; Bell, J.M.; Breiding, M.J.; Xu, L. Traumatic Brain Injury–Related Emergency Department Visits, Hospitalizations, and Deaths—United States, 2007 and 2013. *MMWR Surveill. Summ.* **2017**, *66*, 1–16. [CrossRef]
2. Cassidy, J.D.; Carroll, L.J.; Peloso, P.M.; Borg, J.; von Holst, H.; Holm, L.; Kraus, J.; Coronado, V. Incidence, risk factors and prevention of mild traumatic brain injury: Results of the WHO Collaborating Centre Task Force on Mild Traumatic Brain Injury. *J. Rehabil. Med.* **2004**, *36*, 28–60. [CrossRef]
3. Powell, J.M.; Ferraro, J.V.; Dikmen, S.S.; Temkin, N.R.; Bell, K.R. Accuracy of mild traumatic brain injury diagnosis. *Arch. Phys. Med. Rehabil.* **2008**, *89*, 1550–1555. [CrossRef]
4. Wickwire, E.M.; Williams, S.G.; Roth, T.; Capaldi, V.F.; Jaffe, M.; Moline, M.; Motamedi, G.K.; Morgan, G.W.; Mysliwiec, V.; Germain, A.; et al. Sleep, Sleep Disorders, and Mild Traumatic Brain Injury. What We Know and What We Need to Know: Findings from a National Working Group. *Neurotherapeutics* **2016**, *13*, 403–417. [CrossRef]
5. Mollayeva, T.; Mollayeva, S.; Colantonio, A. The Risk of Sleep Disorder among Persons with Mild Traumatic Brain Injury. *Curr. Neurol. Neurosci. Rep.* **2016**, *16*, 55. [CrossRef]
6. Vermaelen, J.; Greiffenstein, P.; deBoisblanc, B.P. Sleep in traumatic brain injury. *Crit. Care Clinic.* **2015**, *31*, 551–561. [CrossRef]

7. Kraus, M.F.; Susmaras, T.; Caughlin, B.P.; Walker, C.J.; Sweeney, J.A.; Little, D.M. White matter integrity and cognition in chronic traumatic brain injury: A diffusion tensor imaging study. *Brain* **2007**, *130*, 2508–2519. [CrossRef]

8. Viola-Saltzman, M.; Watson, N.F. Traumatic Brain Injury and Sleep Disorders. *Neurol. Clin.* **2012**, *30*, 1299–1312. [CrossRef]

9. Arciniegas, D.B.; Topkoff, J.; Silver, J.M. Neuropsychiatric aspects of traumatic brain injury. *Curr. Treat. Options Neurol.* **2000**, *2*, 169–186. [CrossRef]

10. Orff, H.J.; Ayalon, L.; Drummond, S.P. Traumatic brain injury and sleep disturbance: A review of current research. *J. Head Trauma Rehabil.* **2009**, *24*, 155–165. [CrossRef]

11. Viola-Saltzman, M.; Musleh, C. Traumatic brain injury-induced sleep disorders. *Neuropsychiatr. Dis. Treat.* **2016**, *12*, 339–348. [CrossRef]

12. Gilbert, K.S.; Kark, S.M.; Gehrman, P.; Bogdanova, Y. Sleep Disturbances, TBI and PTSD: Implications for Treatment and Recovery. *Clin. Psychol. Rev.* **2015**, *40*, 195–212. [CrossRef]

13. Yaeger, K.; Alhilali, L.; Fakhran, S. Evaluation of tentorial length and angle in sleep-wake disturbances after mild traumatic brain injury. *Am. J. Roentgenol.* **2014**, *202*, 614–618. [CrossRef]

14. Fakhran, S. Symptomatic white matter changes in mild traumatic brain injury resemble pathologic features of early alzheimer dementia. *Radiology* **2013**, *269*, 249–257. [CrossRef]

15. Hazra, A. Delayed thalamic astrocytosis and disrupted sleep-wake patterns in a preclinical model of traumatic brain injury. *J. Neurosci Res.* **2014**, *92*, 1434–1445. [CrossRef]

16. Shekleton, J.; Parcell, D.L.; Redman, J.R.; Phipps-Nelson, J.; Ponsford, J.L.; Rajaratnam, S.M.W. Sleep disturbance and melatonin levels following traumatic brain injury. *Neurology* **2010**, *74*, 1732–1738. [CrossRef]

17. Wilkinson, C.W.; Pagulayan, K.F.; Petrie, E.C.; Mayer, C.L.; Colasurdo, E.A.; Shofer, J.B.; Hart, K.L.; Hoff, D.; Tarabochia, M.A.; Peskind, E.R. High Prevalence of Chronic Pituitary and Target-Organ Hormone Abnormalities after Blast-Related Mild Traumatic Brain Injury. *Front. Neurol.* **2012**, *3*, 11. [CrossRef]

18. Zeitzer, J.M.; Friedman, L.; O'Hara, R. Insomnia in the context of traumatic brain injury. *J. Rehabil. Res. Dev.* **2009**, *46*, 827–836. [CrossRef]

19. Sabir, M.; Gaudreault, P.O.; Freyburger, M.; Massart, R.; Blanchet-Cohen, A.; Jaber, M.; Gosselin, N.; Mongrain, V. Impact of traumatic brain injury on sleep structure, electrocorticographic activity and transcriptome in mice. *Brain Behav. Immun.* **2015**, *47*, 118–130. [CrossRef]

20. Hong, C.T.; Wong, C.S.; Ma, H.P.; Wu, D.; Huang, Y.H.; Wu, C.C.; Lin, C.M.; Su, Y.K.; Liao, K.H.; Ou, J.C.; et al. PERIOD3 polymorphism is associated with sleep quality recovery after a mild traumatic brain injury. *J. Neurol. Sci.* **2015**, *358*, 385–389. [CrossRef]

21. El Shakankiry, H.M. Sleep physiology and sleep disorders in childhood. *Nat. Sci. Sleep* **2011**, *3*, 101–114. [CrossRef]

22. Schreiber, S.; Barkai, G.; Gur-Hartman, T.; Peles, E.; Tov, N.; Dolberg, O.T.; Pick, C.G. Long-lasting sleep patterns of adult patients with minor traumatic brain injury (mTBI) and non-mTBI subjects. *Sleep Med.* **2008**, *9*, 481–487. [CrossRef] [PubMed]

23. Lucke-Wold, B.P.; Smith, K.E.; Nguyen, L.; Turner, R.C.; Logsdon, A.F.; Jackson, G.J.; Huber, J.D.; Rosen, C.L.; Miller, D.B. Sleep disruption and the sequelae associated with traumatic brain injury. *Neurosci. Biobehav. Rev.* **2015**, *55*, 68–77. [CrossRef] [PubMed]

24. Kaufman, Y.; Tzischinsky, O.; Epstein, R.; Etzioni, A.; Lavie, P.; Pillar, G. Long-term sleep disturbances in adolescents after minor head injury. *Pediatr. Neurol.* **2001**, *24*, 129–134. [CrossRef]

25. Ouellet, M.C.; Morin, C.M. Subjective and objective measures of insomnia in the context of traumatic brain injury: A preliminary study. *Sleep Med.* **2006**, *7*, 486–497. [CrossRef] [PubMed]

26. Waldron-Perrine, B.; McGuire, A.P.; Spencer, R.J.; Drag, L.L.; Pangilinan, P.H.; Bieliauskas, L.A. The influence of sleep and mood on cognitive functioning among veterans being evaluated for mild traumatic brain injury. *Mil. Med.* **2012**, *177*, 1293–1301. [CrossRef] [PubMed]

27. Bolge, S.C.; Doan, J.F.; Kannan, H.; Baran, R.W. Association of insomnia with quality of life, work productivity, and activity impairment. *Qual. Life Res.* **2009**, *18*, 415–422. [CrossRef] [PubMed]

28. Mathias, J.; Alvaro, P. Prevalence of sleep disturbances, disorders and problems following traumatic brain injury: A meta-analysis. *Sleep Med.* **2017**, *13*, 898–905. [CrossRef] [PubMed]

29. Ouellet, M.C.; Beaulieu-Bonneau, S.; Morin, C.M. Insomnia in patients with traumatic brain injury: Frequency, characteristics, and risk factors. *J. Head Trauma Rehabil.* **2006**, *21*, 199–212. [CrossRef] [PubMed]

30. Sullivan, K.A.; Berndt, S.L.; Edmed, S.L.; Smith, S.S.; Allan, A.C. Poor sleep predicts subacute postconcussion symptoms following mild traumatic brain injury. *Appl. Neuropsychol. Adult* **2016**, *23*, 426–435. [CrossRef]

31. Ouellet, M.C.; Savard, J.; Morin, C.M. Insomnia following Traumatic Brain Injury: A Review. *Neurorehabil. Neural Repair* **2004**, *18*, 187–198. [CrossRef] [PubMed]

32. Ohayon, M.M. Epidemiology of insomnia: What we know and what we still need to learn. *Sleep Med. Rev.* **2002**, *6*, 97–111. [CrossRef] [PubMed]

33. Fichtenberg, N.L.; Millis, S.R.; Mann, N.R.; Zafonte, R.D.; Millard, A.E. Factors associated with insomnia among post-acute traumatic brain injury survivors. *Brain Inj.* **2000**, *14*, 659–667. [CrossRef] [PubMed]

34. Tham, S.W.; Fales, J.; Palermo, T.M. Subjective and objective assessment of sleep in adolescents with mild traumatic brain injury. *J. Neurotrauma* **2015**, *32*, 847–852. [CrossRef] [PubMed]

35. Hu, T.; Hunt, C.; Ouchterlony, D. Is Age Associated With the Severity of Post-Mild Traumatic Brain Injury Symptoms? *Can. J. Neurol. Sci.* **2017**, *44*, 384–390. [CrossRef] [PubMed]

36. Petraglia, A.L.; Plog, B.A.; Dayawansa, S.; Chen, M.; Dashnaw, M.L.; Czerniecka, K.; Huang, J.H. The Spectrum of Neurobehavioral Sequelae after Repetitive Mild Traumatic Brain Injury: A Novel Mouse Model of Chronic Traumatic Encephalopathy. *J. Neurotrauma* **2014**, *31*, 1211–1224. [CrossRef] [PubMed]

37. Bryan, C.J. Repetitive traumatic brain injury (or concussion) increases severity of sleep disturbance among deployed military personnel. *Sleep* **2013**, *36*, 941–946. [CrossRef] [PubMed]

38. McKee, A.C.; Robinson, M.E. Military-related traumatic brain injury and neurodegeneration. *Alzheimers Dement.* **2014**, *10*, 242–253. [CrossRef] [PubMed]

39. Hicks, R.R.; Fertig, S.J.; Desrocher, R.E.; Koroshetz, W.J.; Pancrazio, J.J. Neurological effects of blast injury. *J. Trauma* **2010**, *68*, 1257–1263. [CrossRef] [PubMed]

40. Sayer, N.A.; Chiros, C.E.; Sigford, B.; Scott, S.; Clothier, B.; Pickett, T.; Lew, H.L. Characteristics and Rehabilitation Outcomes among Patients with Blast and Other Injuries Sustained During the Global War on Terror. *Arch. Phys. Med. Rehabil.* **2008**, *89*, 163–170. [CrossRef]

41. Linton, S.J.; Bryngelsson, I.L. Insomnia and its relationship to work and health in a working-age population. *J. Occup. Rehabil.* **2000**, *10*, 169–183. [CrossRef]

42. Baumann, C.R.; Werth, E.; Stocker, R.; Ludwig, S.; Bassetti, C.L. Sleep-wake disturbances 6 months after traumatic brain injury: A prospective study. *Brain* **2007**, *130*, 1873–1883. [CrossRef]

43. Farrell-Carnahan, L.; Barnett, S.; Lamberty, G.; Hammond, F.M.; Kretzmer, T.S.; Franke, L.M.; Geiss, M.; Howe, L.; Nakase-Richardson, R. Insomnia symptoms and behavioural health symptoms in veterans 1 year after traumatic brain injury. *Brain Inj.* **2015**, *29*, 1400–1408. [CrossRef] [PubMed]

44. Losoi, H.; Silverberg, N.D.; Wäljas, M.; Turunen, S.; Rosti-Otajärvi, E.; Helminen, M.; Luoto, T.M.; Julkunen, J.; Öhman, J.; Iverson, G.L. Recovery from Mild Traumatic Brain Injury in Previously Healthy Adults. *J. Neurotrauma* **2016**, *33*, 766–776. [CrossRef] [PubMed]

45. McMahon, P.J.; Hricik, A.; Yue, J.K.; Puccio, A.M.; Inoue, T.; Lingsma, H.F.; Vassar, M.J. Symptomatology and functional outcome in mild traumatic brain injury: Results from the prospective TRACK-TBI study. *J. Neurotrauma* **2014**, *31*, 26–33. [CrossRef]

46. Ma, H.P.; Ou, J.C.; Yeh, C.T.; Wu, D.; Tsai, S.H.; Chiu, W.T.; Hu, C.J. Recovery from sleep disturbance precedes that of depression and anxiety following mild traumatic brain injury: A 6-week follow-up study. *BMJ Open* **2014**, *4*. [CrossRef] [PubMed]

47. Martindale, S.L.; Farrell-Carnahan, L.V.; Ulmer, C.S.; Kimbrel, N.A.; McDonald, S.D.; Rowland, J.A. VA Mid-Atlantic MIRECC Registry Workgroup. Sleep Quality in Returning Veterans: The Influence of Mild Traumatic Brain Injury. *Rehabil. Psychol.* **2017**, *62*, 563–570. [CrossRef]

48. Theadom, A.; Starkey, N.; Jones, K.; Cropley, M.; Parmar, P.; Barker-Collo, S.; Feigin, V.L. Sleep difficulties and their impact on recovery following mild traumatic brain injury in children. *Brain Inj.* **2016**, *30*, 1243–1248. [CrossRef] [PubMed]

49. Pillar, G.; Averbooch, E.; Katz, N.; Peled, N.; Kaufman, Y.; Shahar, E. Prevalence and risk of sleep disturbances in adolescents after minor head injury. *Pediatr. Neurol.* **2003**, *29*, 131–135. [CrossRef]

50. Theadom, A.; Parag, V.; Dowell, T.; McPherson, K.; Starkey, N.; Barker-Collo, S.; Jones, K.; Ameratunga, S.; Feigin, V.L. Persistent problems 1 year after mild traumatic brain injury: A longitudinal population study in New Zealand. *Br. J. Gen. Pract.* **2015**, *66*, 16–23. [CrossRef]

51. Duclos, C.; Beauregard, M.P.; Bottari, C.; Ouellet, M.C.; Gosselin, N. The impact of poor sleep on cognition and activities of daily living after traumatic brain injury: A review. *Aust. Occup. Ther. J.* **2015**, *62*, 2–12. [CrossRef] [PubMed]

52. Theadom, A.; Cropley, M.; Parmar, P.; Barker-Collo, S.; Starkey, N.; Jones, K.; Feigin, V.L. BIONIC Research Group. Sleep difficulties one year following mild traumatic brain injury in a population-based study. *Sleep Med.* **2015**, *16*, 926–932. [CrossRef] [PubMed]

53. Bonneau, S.B.; Ouellet, M.C. Fatigue in the first year after traumatic brain injury: Course, relationship with injury severity, and correlates. *Neuropsychol. Rehabil.* **2017**, *27*, 983–1001. [CrossRef] [PubMed]

54. Wylie, G.R.; Flashman, L.A. Understanding the interplay between mild traumatic brain injury and cognitive fatigue: Models and treatments. *Concussion* **2017**, *2*, 50. [CrossRef] [PubMed]

55. Norre, J.; Heitger, M.; Leathem, J.; Anderson, T.; Jones, R.; Flett, R. Mild traumatic brain injury and fatigue: A prospective longitudinal study. *Brain Inj.* **2010**, *24*, 1528–1538. [CrossRef] [PubMed]

56. Stulemeijer, M.; van der Werf, S.; Bleijenberg, G.; Biert, J.; Brauer, J.; Vos, P. Recovery from mild traumatic brain injury: A focus on fatigue. *J. Neurol.* **2006**, *253*, 1041–1047. [CrossRef] [PubMed]

57. Albicini, M.S.; Lee, J.; McKinlay, A. Ongoing daytime behavioural problems in university students following childhood mild traumatic brain injury. *Int. J. Rehabil. Res.* **2016**, *39*, 77–83. [CrossRef]

58. Mollayeva, T.; Pratt, B.; Mollayeva, S.; Shapiro, C.M.; Cassidy, J.D.; Colantonio, A. The relationship between insomnia and disability in workers with mild traumatic brain injury/concussion: Insomnia and disability in chronic mild traumatic brain injury. *Sleep Med.* **2016**, *20*, 157–166. [CrossRef]

59. Lavigne, G.; Khoury, S.; Chauny, J.M.; Desautels, A. Pain and sleep in post-concussion/mild traumatic brain injury. *Pain* **2015**, *156*, 75–85. [CrossRef]

60. Suzuki, Y.; Khoury, S.; El-Khatib, H.; Chauny, J.M.; Paquet, J.; Giguère, J.F.; Denis, R.; Gosselin, N.; Lavigne, G.J.; Arbour, C. Individuals with pain need more sleep in the early stage of mild traumatic brain injury. *Sleep Med.* **2017**, *33*, 36–42. [CrossRef]

61. MacGregor, A.J.; Dougherty, A.L.; Tang, J.J.; Galarneau, M.R. Postconcussive symptom reporting among US combat veterans with mild traumatic brain injury from Operation Iraqi Freedom. *J. Head Trauma Rehabil.* **2013**, *28*, 59–67. [CrossRef] [PubMed]

62. Sherman, K.B.; Goldberg, M.; Bell, K.R. Traumatic Brain Injury and Pain. *Phys. Med. Rehabil. Clin. N. Am.* **2006**, *17*, 473–490. [CrossRef] [PubMed]

63. Sandsmark, D.K.; Elliott, J.E.; Lim, M.M. Sleep-Wake Disturbances after Traumatic Brain Injury: Synthesis of Human and Animal Studies. *Sleep* **2017**, *40*. [CrossRef] [PubMed]

64. Tregear, S.; Reston, J.; Schoelles, K.; Phillips, B. Obstructive sleep apnea and risk of motor vehicle crash: Systematic review and meta-analysis. *J. Clin. Sleep Med.* **2009**, *5*, 573–581. [PubMed]

65. Howlett, J.R.; Stein, M.B. Post-Traumatic Stress Disorder: Relationship to Traumatic Brain Injury and Approach to Treatment. In *Translation Research in Traumatic Brain Injury (Frontiers in Neuroscience)*, 1st ed.; Laskowitz, D., Grant, G., Eds.; CRC Press/Taylor and Francis Group: Boca Raton, FL, USA, 2016; Volume 57, Chapter 16; ISBN 978-1-4665-8491-4.

66. Tanev, K.S.; Pentel, K.Z.; Kredlow, M.A.; Charney, M.E. PTSD and TBI co-morbidity: Scope, clinical presentation and treatment options. *Brain Inj.* **2014**, *28*, 261–270. [CrossRef] [PubMed]

67. Capaldi, V.F.; Guerrero, M.L.; Killgore, W.D. Sleep disruptions among returning combat veterans from Iraq and Afghanistan. *Mil. Med.* **2011**, *176*, 879–888. [CrossRef]

68. Ayalon, L.; Borodkin, K.; Dishon, L.; Kanety, H.; Dagan, Y. Circadian rhythm sleep disorders following mild traumatic brain injury. *Neurology* **2007**, *68*, 1136–1140. [CrossRef]

69. Roth, T. Prevalence, associated risks, and treatment patterns of insomnia. *J. Clin. Psychiatry* **2005**, *6*, 10–13.

70. Capaldi, V.F.; Kim, J.R.; Grillakis, A.A.; Taylor, M.R.; York, C.M. Insomnia in the Military: Application and Effectiveness of Cognitive and Pharmacologic Therapies. *Curr. Psychiatry Rep.* **2015**, *17*, 85. [CrossRef]

71. Blinman, T.A.; Houseknecht, E.; Snyder, C.; Wiebe, D.J.; Nance, M.L. Postconcussive symptoms in hospitalized pediatric patients after mild traumatic brain injury. *J. Pediatr. Surg.* **2009**, *44*, 1223–1228. [CrossRef]

72. Bogdanov, S.; Naismith, S.; Lah, S. Sleep outcomes following sleep-hygiene-related interventions for individuals with traumatic brain injury: A systematic review. *Brain Inj.* **2017**, *31*, 422–433. [CrossRef] [PubMed]

73. Ouellet, M.C.; Morin, C.M. Efficacy of cognitive-behavioral therapy for insomnia associated with traumatic brain injury: A single-case experimental design. *Arch. Phys. Med. Rehabil.* **2007**, *88*, 1581–1592. [CrossRef] [PubMed]

74. Nguyen, S.; McKay, A.; Wong, D.; Rajaratnam, S.M.; Spitz, G.; Williams, G.; Mansfield, D.; Ponsford, J.L. Cognitive Behavior Therapy to Treat Sleep Disturbance and Fatigue After Traumatic Brain Injury: A Pilot Randomized Controlled Trial. *Arch. Phys. Med. Rehabil.* **2017**, *98*, 1508–1517. [CrossRef] [PubMed]

75. Luik, A.I.; Kyle, S.D.; Espie, C.A. Digital Cognitive Behavioral Therapy (dCBT) for Insomnia: A State-of-the-Science Review. *Curr. Sleep Med. Rep.* **2017**, *3*, 48–56. [CrossRef] [PubMed]

76. Espie, C.A.; Luik, A.I.; Cape, J.; Drake, C.L.; Siriwardena, A.N.; Ong, J.C.; Gordon, C.; Bostock, S.; Bostock, S.; Hames, P.; et al. Digital Cognitive Behavioural Therapy for Insomnia versus sleep hygiene education: The impact of improved sleep on functional health, quality of life and psychological well-being. Study protocol for a randomised controlled trial. *Trials* **2016**, *17*, 257. [CrossRef]

77. Sirdifield, C.; Chipchase, S.Y.; Owen, S.; Siriwardena, A.N. A Systematic Review and Meta-Synthesis of Patients' Experiences and Perceptions of Seeking and Using Benzodiazepines and Z-Drugs: Towards Safer Prescribing. *Patient* **2017**, *10*, 1–15. [CrossRef] [PubMed]

78. Larson, E.B.; Zollman, F.S. The effect of sleep medications on cognitive recovery from traumatic brain injury. *J. Head Trauma Rehabil.* **2010**, *25*, 61–67. [CrossRef]

79. Hajak, G.; Muller, W.E.; Wittchen, H.U.; Pittrow, D.; Kirch, W. Abuse and dependence potential for the non-benzodiazepine hypnotics zolpidem and zopiclone: A review of case reports and epidemiological data. *Addiction* **2003**, *98*, 1371–1378. [CrossRef]

80. Li Pi Shan, R.S.; Ashworth, N.L. Comparison of lorazapam and zopicloine for insomnia in patients with stroke and brain injury. *Am. J. Phys. Med. Rehabil.* **2004**, *83*, 421–427. [CrossRef]

81. Glenn, M.B.; Wroblewski, B. Twenty years of pharmacology. *J. Head Trauma Rehabil.* **2005**, *20*, 51–61. [CrossRef]

82. Grima, N.A.; Rajaratam, S.M.W.; Mansfield, D.; Sletten, T.L.; Spitz, G.; Ponsford, J.L. Efficacy of melatonin for sleep disturbance following traumatic brain injury: A randomized controlled trial. *BMC Med.* **2018**, *16*, 8. [CrossRef] [PubMed]

83. Leguerica, A.; Jasey, N.; Portelli Tremont, J.N.; Chiaravalloti, N.D. Pilot study on the effect of ramelteon on sleep disturbance after traumatic brain injury: Preliminary evidence from a clinical trial. *Arch. Phys. Med. Rehabil.* **2015**, *96*, 1802–1809. [CrossRef] [PubMed]

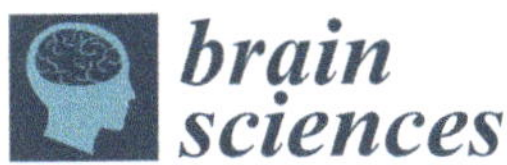 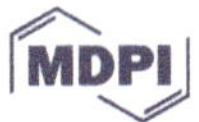

Article

Sleep Disorders Following Mild and Moderate Traumatic Brain Injury

Laith Thamer Al-Ameri [1,*], **Talib Saddam Mohsin** [1] **and Ali Tarik Abdul Wahid** [2]

1   Al-Kindy College of Medicine, University of Baghdad, Baghdad, Iraq; talib.almuhsin@gmail.com
2   College of Medicine, University of Baghdad, Baghdad, Iraq; azdh_1978@yahoo.com
*   Correspondence: laith.thamer@yahoo.com; Tel.: +964-770-534-3467

Received: 27 November 2018; Accepted: 10 January 2019; Published: 11 January 2019

Abstract: (1) Background: Sleeping disorders are frequently reported following traumatic brain injury (TBI). Different forms of sleeping disorders have been reported, such as sleepiness, insomnia, changes in sleeping latency, and others. (2) Methods: A case-control study with 62 patients who were victims of mild or moderate TBI with previous admissions to Iraqi tertiary neurosurgical centers were enrolled as the first group, and 158 patients with no history of trauma were considered as the control. All were 18 years of age or older, and the severity of the trauma and sleep disorders was assessed. The Pittsburgh sleep quality index was used to assess sleep disorders with average need for sleep per day and average sleep latency were assessed in both groups. Chi-square and t-test calculations were used to compare different variables. (3) Results: 39 patients (24.7%) of the controlled group experienced sleeping disorders compared to TBI group with 45 patients (72.6%), *P*-value < 0.00001. A total of 42 patients were diagnosed on admission as having a mild degree of TBI (mean GCS 13.22 ± 1.76) and 20 patients were diagnosed with moderate TBI (mean GCS11.05 ± 1.14. 27). A total of 27 (46.28%) patients with mild severity TBI and 18 patients (90%) of moderate severity were considered to experience sleeping disorders, *P*-value 0.0339. Each of the mild and moderate TBI subgroups show a *P*-value < 0.00001 compared to the control group. Average sleep hours needed per day for TBI and the control were 8.02 ± 1.04 h and 7.26 ± 0.58 h, respectively, *P*-value < 0.00001. Average sleep latency for the TBI and the control groups were 13.32 ± 3.16 min and 13.93 ± 3.07 min respectively, *P*-value 0.065. (4) Conclusion: Sleep disturbances are more common following mild and moderate TBI three months after the injury with more hours needed for sleep per day and no significant difference in sleep latency. Sleep disturbances increase in frequency with the increase in the severity of TBI.

Keywords: traumatic brain injury; sleep disorders; sleep latency

---

1. Introduction

Sleep disorders frequently follow a traumatic brain injury (TBI), with reports of 30%–70% of TBI patients experiencing negative impacts on quality of life and rehabilitation [1–5]. Sleep disorders have been shown to aggravate psychiatric problems, affect the mood and behavior of injured patients, and thus contribute to poor neuronal remodeling following the injury [6,7]. Different patterns of sleep disorders have been reported, such as hypersomnia, insomnia, change in sleep latency, narcolepsy, and parasomnia. [4,6–8].

Many factors contribute to sleep disorders, with brain trauma itself being the most important, including primary and secondary effects. A primary effect results from direct injury to brain tissues through acceleration-deceleration forces and/or rotational forces with consequent diffuse axonal injury, while secondary effects results from cellular events caused by hypoxia and raised intracranial pressure [9].

Specific locations of brain injury may be responsible for specific patterns of sleeping disorders. Thalamic and caudal midbrain injury may be responsible for hypersomnia, while direct injury impact on the pineal gland and tentorium may result in insomnia due to the effect on melatonin homeostasis [2,4,10–12].

Another hypothesis states that supra-chiasmatic damage may result in a consequent disturbance in the circadian rhythm, with a mixed picture of insomnia and hypersomnia [4].

Rather than factors related to brain trauma itself, sleep disorders may be a result of neuropsychiatric conditions, such as anxiety or depression, or a result of pain due to associated musculoskeletal trauma or spasm. Anxiety, depression, and pain are considered to be comorbidity factors associated with sleep disorders following TBI [4,13,14].

Traumatic brain injury is a leading cause of death and disability, with different etiologies, types, and severity. Different patterns of complications and outcomes vary widely according to the severity of TBI [15,16]. The severity is assessed by the Glasgow Coma Scale (GCS) based on the level of consciousness, with the TBI being classified into mild (GCS 15-13), moderate (12-9), or severe (8 or less) [15,17].

The Pittsburgh sleep quality index (PSQI) is used to assess sleep disorders and shows good reliability and validity in both young and old age groups [18–20]. The PSQI has been translated into the Arabic language successfully, showing acceptable reliability and validity [21].

Our study aimed to evaluate sleep disorders in patients with previous mild and moderate TBI that were admitted to tertiary neurosurgical centers in Baghdad, Iraq. It is one of the first studies conducted on patients attending Iraqi tertiary neurosurgical centers and clinic to consult for such a reason.

2. Materials and Methods

This is a case-control study with 220 patients enrolled; 62 of them were victims of mild or moderate TBI (three months post-injury) who previously attended tertiary neurosurgical centers in Baghdad, Iraq, and 158 patients had no history regarding TBI, considered to be the control group. The TBI patients were with different etiologies, including falling from a height, road traffic accidents, and being hit by an object, and all presented with no persistent neurological deficit. Age and sex was matched between both groups. Of the TBI group, 42 out of 62 suffered a mild TBI while the other 20 patients were considered to have moderate TBI. Severity determination of the TBI was based on assessment through the GCS. All participants in both groups were 18 years or older. Patients of the TBI group with sleeping disorders or psychiatric disorders prior to the injury were excluded from the study. The exclusion criteria of the control group were patients with psychiatric illnesses, previous TBI, or those who were on hypnotics.

Admission GCS scores were obtained from the patients' records, while sleep disorders were assessed through the PSQI translated to the Arabic language for self-reporting sleep quality. The PSQI were administered to patients three months following the TBI. Global scoring was undertaken for patients in both groups to assess the presence of sleep disorder, with the assessment including the average need for sleep per day and average sleep latency. The global PSQI score is calculated by totaling the seven component scores, providing an overall score ranging from 0 to 21, where a lower score denotes a healthier sleep quality. Traditionally, the items from the PSQI have been summed to create a total score to measure overall sleep quality. A total score of 5 or greater indicates poor sleep quality, and a score lower than 5 is regarded as normal.

Statistical analysis was completed with data introduced to IBM SPSS 22 software (Chicago, IL, USA). Chi-square and t-test calculations were used to compare different variables with a P-value < 0.05 considered significant. Normality of distribution of dependent variables was checked through application of Shapiro–Wilk, Levene's test was used to find out homogeneity of dependent variables variances.

Ethical and scientific approval was obtained from the scientific unit at Al-Kindy College of Medicine, University of Baghdad. Written consent was obtained from each participant enrolled in the study after clarification to them of the purpose of the study.

3. Results

Data was collected from both groups and analyzed using a Chi-square and *t*-test. The male to female ratio was 4:1, with a mean age of 35 ± 14 years. Mean age for TBI group was 36.3 ± 14.94, while mean age for control group was 34.59 ± 13.8, see Tables 1 and 2. A total of 39 patients (24.7%) of the control group experienced sleeping disorders according to the PSQI, and 119 did not, while 45 patients (72.6%) of the TBI group experienced sleeping disorders and 17 patients did not. *P*-value was <0.00001, see Table 3.

Table 1. Difference between mean and standard deviation of age of studied personnel according to the groups.

Group	*N*	Mean Age	Standard Deviation	*P*-Value
Traumatic brain injury (TBI) group	62	36.3065	14.94755	0.418
Control	158	34.5886	13.80950	

Table 2. Difference between mean and standard deviation of gender of studied personnel.

Gender	*N*	Mean	Standard Deviation	*P*-Value
male	165	1.7212	0.44977	0.863
female	55	1.7091	0.45837	

Table 3. Data for traumatic brain injury (TBI) and the control groups.

	TBI	Control	*P*-Value	Test Value	*df*	Method
Sleep disorders (No. of patients)	45 (72.6%)	39 (24.7%)	$P < 0.0001$	43.278 χ^2 value		Chi-square
Sleep hours/day *	7. 94± 1.07	7.26 ± 0.58	$P < 0.0001$	4.72 *t* value	218	*t*-test
Sleep latency (min) *	13.22 ± 3.16	13.93 ± 3.07	P 0.131	1.517 *t* value	218	*t*-test

* mean ± standard deviation.

Of the TBI group, 42 patients were diagnosed on admission as having a mild degree of TBI, with a mean GCS score of 13.22 ± 1.76. A total of 20 patients were diagnosed as having a moderate TBI, with a mean GCS score of 11.05 ± 1.14. Both subgroups were triaged as having TBI by a neurosurgical on call trauma team. Of these subgroups, 27 patients (46.28%) of mild severity TBI and 18 patients (90%) of moderate severity experienced sleeping disorders according to the PSQI. Comparing both subgroups (mild and moderate TBI) showed a *P*-value of 0.0339. Each of mild and moderate TBI subgroups showed a *P*-value <0.00001 compared to the control group, see Table 4.

Table 4. Data for mild and moderate traumatic brain injury (TBI) subgroups.

	Mild TBI	Moderate TBI	*P*-Value	Method
Initial GCS	13.22 ± 1.76	11.05 ± 1.14		
Sleep disorders (No. of patients)	27 (64.28%)	18 (90%)	0.0339 χ^2 4.501	Chi-square

The average sleep hours needed per day was assessed for patients in the TBI and control groups, with means of 8.02 ± 1.04 h and 7.26 ± 0.58 h, respectively. *P*-value < 0.00001, Table 3.

The average sleep latency was assessed for patients in the TBI and control groups, with means of 13.32 ± 3.16 min and 13.93 ± 3.07 min, respectively. *P*-value 0.065, Table 3.

4. Discussion

Sleep disturbances were more common in the TBI group than the control group, with a highly significant *P*-value < 0.00001. A total of 72.6% of the TBI group experienced sleep disturbances, compared to 24.7% in the control group. Sleep disturbances following TBI have been reported frequently in many previous studies when compared to controls. Sleep disturbances in previous studies have, however, shown different pictures. Baumann et al. in 2007 showed 72% of people experienced sleep disturbances following a TBI [6]. Others showed rates that varied widely from 30% to 84% [22]. The extremely high rate obtained in our results may be explained by poor rehabilitation following TBIs in our area.

Different pictures were also shown according to the severity of TBI. Our study assessed sleep disturbances in both mild and moderate groups, separately. The mild TBI and moderate TBI groups showed 46.28% and 90% sleep disturbances rates, respectively. Both had a highly significant *P*-value compared to the control groups (*P*-value < 0.00001); the moderate TBI group had a higher rate than the mild TBI group, with a significant *P*-value of 0.0339. These results are in agreement with the hypothesis stating that sleep disturbances are caused by neuronal damage, such as the damage caused by primary or secondary brain injuries leading to diffuse axonal injury affecting sleep-regulating regions. This type of damage is expected to be greater the more severe the TBI is [4,5].

Our study shows that more hours are needed for sleep per day in the TBI group compared with the control group, with a mean average hours of 8.02 ± 1.04 and 7.26 ± 0.58, respectively. The *P*-value was highly significant (*P* < 0.00001). These results agree with others, including Lukas et al. who showed similar result of 8.3 ± 1.1 versus 7.1 ± 0.8 h for the TBI group and the control, respectively, with high significance (*P* < 0.00001) [5].

Concerning sleep latency, although the TBI group was lower than the control group at 13.93 ± 3.07 and 13.22 ± 3.16, respectively, the difference was not significant between the TBI and control groups, with a *P*-value of 0.065. Lukas et al. demonstrate significant difference in sleep latency, with a *P*-value of 0.0009 [5]. However, in their meta-analysis, Grima et al. [3] showed no difference in sleep latency when comparing different studies. They did find shorter sleep latency to REM sleep, however this was not analyzed in our study due to laboratory limitations.

Limitations of the study include small sample size, the fact that patients were from centers in Baghdad City only, and the unavailability of well-equipped sleep laboratories. Further studies are needed to include all Iraqi governorates.

5. Conclusions

Sleep disturbances are common in patients following mild and moderate TBI three months after the injury. More hours are needed for sleep per day in previous TBI patients versus the general population. There is no significant change in sleep latency. Sleep disturbances increase in frequency with the increase in the severity of the TBI assessed by the GCS.

Author Contributions: L.T. draft and revise the manuscript; T.S.M., revision of the statistics, revision of the results, revision of PSQI data; A.T.A.W., collection of additional data for same patients from records, assembly of these data, participate in final revision.

Funding: This research received no external funding.

Acknowledgments: We would like to thank Ahmed Abed Marzook for his contribution in statistical analysis.

Conflicts of Interest: The authors declare no conflict of interest.

References

1. Ponsford, J.; Parcell, D.; Sinclair, K.; Roper, M.; Rajaratnam, S. Changes in Sleep Patterns Following Traumatic Brain Injury. *Neurorehabil. Neural. Repair.* **2013**, *27*, 613–621. [CrossRef] [PubMed]
2. Shekleton, J.; Parcell, D.; Redman, J.; Phipps-Nelson, J.; Ponsford, J.; Rajaratnam, S. Sleep disturbance and melatonin levels following traumatic brain injury. *Neurology* **2010**, *74*, 1732–1738. [CrossRef] [PubMed]

3. Grima, N.; Ponsford, J.; Rajaratnam, S.; Mansfield, D.; Pase, M. Sleep Disturbances in Traumatic Brain Injury: A Meta-Analysis. *J. Clin. Sleep Med.* **2016**, *12*, 419–428. [CrossRef] [PubMed]

4. Viola-Saltzman, M.; Musleh, C. Traumatic brain injury-induced sleep disorders. *Neuropsychiatr. Dis. Treat.* **2016**, *12*, 339. [CrossRef] [PubMed]

5. Imbach, L.L.; Valko, P.O.; Li, T.; Maric, A.; Symeonidou, E.R.; Stover, J.F.; Bassetti, C.L.; Mica, L.; Werth, E.; Baumann, C.R. Increased sleep need and daytime sleepiness 6 months after traumatic brain injury: A prospective controlled clinical trial. *Brain* **2015**, *138*, 726–735. [CrossRef] [PubMed]

6. Baumann, C.; Werth, E.; Stocker, R.; Ludwig, S.; Bassetti, C. Sleep-wake disturbances 6 months after traumatic brain injury: A prospective study. *Brain* **2007**, *130*, 1873–1883. [CrossRef] [PubMed]

7. Rao, V.; Rollings, P. Sleep disturbances following traumatic brain injury. *Curr. Treat. Opt. Neurol.* **2002**, *4*, 77–87. [CrossRef]

8. Castriotta, R.; Murthy, J. Sleep Disorders in Patients with Traumatic Brain Injury. *CNS Drugs* **2011**, *25*, 175–185. [CrossRef] [PubMed]

9. Andriessen, T.; Jacobs, B.; Vos, P. Clinical characteristics and pathophysiological mechanisms of focal and diffuse traumatic brain injury. *J. Cell Mol. Med.* **2010**, *14*, 2381–2392. [CrossRef] [PubMed]

10. Kemp, S.; Biswas, R.; Neumann, V.; Coughlan, A. The value of melatonin for sleep disorders occurring post-head injury: A pilot RCT. *Brain Inj.* **2004**, *18*, 911–919. [CrossRef]

11. Yaeger, K.; Alhilali, L.; Fakhran, S. Evaluation of Tentorial Length and Angle in Sleep-Wake Disturbances After Mild Traumatic Brain Injury. *AJR Am. J. Roentgenol.* **2014**, *202*, 614–618. [CrossRef] [PubMed]

12. Llompart-Pou, J.A.; Pérez, G.; Raurich, J.M.; Riesco, M.; Brell, M.; Ibáñez, J.; Pérez-Bárcena, J.; Abadal, J.M.; Homar, J.; Burguera, B. Loss of Cortisol Circadian Rhythm in Patients with Traumatic Brain Injury: A Microdialysis Evaluation. *Neurocrit. Care* **2010**, *13*, 211–216. [CrossRef] [PubMed]

13. Viola-Saltzman, M.; Watson, N. Traumatic Brain Injury and Sleep Disorders. *Neurol. Clin.* **2012**, *30*, 1299–1312. [CrossRef]

14. Wiseman-Hakes, C.; Murray, B.J.; Mollayeva, T.; Gargaro, J.; Colantonio, A. A Profile of Sleep Architecture and Sleep Disorders in Adults with Chronic Traumatic Brain Injury. *J. Sleep Disord. Ther.* **2015**, *5*, 224. [CrossRef]

15. Dinsmore, J. Traumatic brain injury: An evidence-based review of management. *Continuing Educ. Anaesth. Crit. Care Pain* **2013**, *13*, 189–195. [CrossRef]

16. Maas, A.; Stocchetti, N.; Bullock, R. Moderate and severe traumatic brain injury in adults. *Lancet Neurol.* **2008**, *7*, 728–741. [CrossRef]

17. Yates, P.; Williams, W.; Harris, A.; Round, A.; Jenkins, R. An epidemiological study of head injuries in a UK population attending an emergency department. *J. Neurol. Neurosurg. Psychiatry* **2006**, *77*, 699–701. [CrossRef] [PubMed]

18. Mondal, P.; Gjevre, J.A.; Taylor-Gjevre, R.M.; Lim, H.J. Relationship between the Pittsburgh Sleep Quality Index and the Epworth Sleepiness Scale in a sleep laboratory referral population. *Nat. Sci. Sleep* **2013**, *5*, 15–21.

19. Spira, A.; Beaudreau, S.; Stone, K.; Kezirian, E.; Lui, L.; Redline, S.; Ancoli-Israel, S.; Ensrud, K.; Stewart, A. Reliability and Validity of the Pittsburgh Sleep Quality Index and the Epworth Sleepiness Scale in Older Men. *J. Gerontol. A Biol. Sci. Med. Sci.* **2011**, *67*, 433–439. [CrossRef]

20. De la Vega, R.; Tomé-Pires, C.; Solé, E.; Racine, M.; Castarlenas, E.; Jensen, M.; Miró, J. The Pittsburgh Sleep Quality Index: Validity and factor structure in young people. *Psychol. Assess.* **2015**, *27*, e22–e27. [CrossRef]

21. Suleiman, K.; Yates, B.; Berger, A.; Pozehl, B.; Meza, J. Translating the Pittsburgh Sleep Quality Index Into Arabic. *West J. Nurs. Res.* **2009**, *32*, 250–268. [CrossRef] [PubMed]

22. Zeitzer, J.; Friedman, L.; OHara, R. Insomnia in the context of traumatic brain injury. *J. Rehabil. Res. Dev.* **2009**, *46*, 827. [CrossRef] [PubMed]

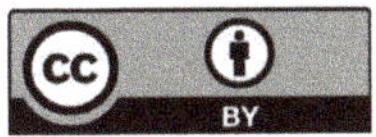

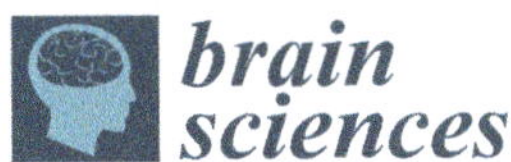 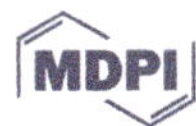

Review

Co-Morbid Insomnia and Sleep Apnea (COMISA): Prevalence, Consequences, Methodological Considerations, and Recent Randomized Controlled Trials

Alexander Sweetman [1,*], Leon Lack [2] and Célyne Bastien [3]

[1] The Adelaide Institute for Sleep Health: A Flinders Centre of Research Excellence, Box 6 Mark Oliphant Building, 5 Laffer Drive, Bedford Park, Flinders University, Adelaide 5042, South Australia, Australia
[2] The Adelaide Institute for Sleep Health: A Flinders Centre of Research Excellence, College of Education Psychology and Social Work, Flinders University, Adelaide 5042, South Australia, Australia; leon.lack@flinders.edu.au
[3] School of Psychology, Félix-Antoine-Savard Pavilion, 2325, rue des Bibliothèques, local 1012, Laval University, Quebec City, QC G1V 0A6, Canada; celyne.bastien@psy.ulaval.ca
* Correspondence: alexander.sweetman@flinders.edu.au; Tel.: +61-8-7421-9908

Received: 15 November 2019; Accepted: 10 December 2019; Published: 12 December 2019

Abstract: Co-morbid insomnia and sleep apnea (COMISA) is a highly prevalent and debilitating disorder, which results in additive impairments to patients' sleep, daytime functioning, and quality of life, and complex diagnostic and treatment decisions for clinicians. Although the presence of COMISA was first recognized by Christian Guilleminault and colleagues in 1973, it received very little research attention for almost three decades, until the publication of two articles in 1999 and 2001 which collectively reported a 30%–50% co-morbid prevalence rate, and re-ignited research interest in the field. Since 1999, there has been an exponential increase in research documenting the high prevalence, common characteristics, treatment complexities, and bi-directional relationships of COMISA. Recent trials indicate that co-morbid insomnia symptoms may be treated with cognitive and behavioral therapy for insomnia, to increase acceptance and use of continuous positive airway pressure therapy. Hence, the treatment of COMISA appears to require nuanced diagnostic considerations, and multi-faceted treatment approaches provided by multi-disciplinary teams of psychologists and physicians. In this narrative review, we present a brief overview of the history of COMISA research, describe the importance of measuring and managing insomnia symptoms in the presence of sleep apnea, discuss important methodological and diagnostic considerations for COMISA, and review several recent randomized controlled trials investigating the combination of CBTi and CPAP therapy. We aim to provide clinicians with pragmatic suggestions and tools to identify, and manage this prevalent COMISA disorder in clinical settings, and discuss future avenues of research to progress the field.

Keywords: COMISA; insomnia; obstructive sleep apnea; sleep-disordered breathing; cognitive behavior therapy for insomnia; continuous positive airway pressure

---

1. Introduction

1.1. Insomnia and Obstructive Sleep Apnea

Insomnia and obstructive sleep apnea (OSA) are the two most common sleep disorders, which both include nocturnal sleep disturbances, impairments to daytime functioning, mood, and quality of life, and high healthcare utilization [1]. As this review focuses on patients with co-morbid insomnia and sleep apnea (COMISA), a brief introduction to both insomnia and OSA is provided below.

Insomnia disorder is characterized by frequent and chronic self-reported difficulties initiating sleep, maintaining sleep, and early morning awakenings from sleep, which are associated with impaired daytime functioning, mood, and quality of life [1,2]. Insomnia disorder is thought to result from a combination of pre-disposing, precipitating, and perpetuating factors, and is conceptualized as a self-perpetuating disorder including elevated cognitive and physiological 'hyper-arousal' [3–5]. The estimated prevalence of insomnia varies widely according to diagnostic criteria and specific populations of interest, however it is thought that 6%–10% of the general population suffer from chronic insomnia disorder, which includes clinically significant and frequent nocturnal sleep disturbances and impaired daytime functioning [6,7]. Although cognitive and behavioral therapy for insomnia (CBTi) leads to long-term improvement of insomnia and is the recommended 'first line' insomnia treatment [8–11], a lack of access to CBTi has resulted in the majority of insomnia sufferers receiving prescriptions for sedative-hypnotic medications as the initial and ongoing treatment [12,13].

Alternatively, OSA is characterized by repetitive brief closure (apnea) or narrowing (hypopnea) of the pharyngeal airway during sleep which result in the cessation or reduction of airflow, reduced oxygen saturation, and commonly terminate in post-apneic arousals from sleep, increased sympathetic activity, and the resumption of airflow [1,14,15]. OSA is thought to result from a combination of anatomical (e.g., a narrow pharyngeal airway), and non-anatomical factors (e.g., impaired upper airway muscle function, low arousal threshold, and unstable control of breathing) [16]. The combination of frequent respiratory events and arousals from sleep throughout the night severely fragments sleep architecture, resulting in perceptions of chronically non-restorative sleep, reduced quality of life, excessive daytime sleepiness, and increased risk of motor-vehicle accidents [17–19]. The most common index of OSA presence and severity is the apnea/hypopnea index (AHI), which represents the average number of respiratory events experienced per hour of sleep. Diagnostic criteria for OSA include an AHI of at least five in the presence of an associated complaint/disorder (e.g., insomnia, sleepiness, fatigue, snoring, hypertension, atrial fibrillation, congestive heart failure, etc.), or an AHI of at least 15 [1]. Mild, moderate, and severe OSA are diagnosed according to an AHI of ≥5 to <15, ≥15 to <30, and ≥30, respectively [15]. The prevalence of OSA varies by diagnostic criteria and the sample population, however it is estimated that approximately 10% of the general population fulfil diagnostic criteria for OSA [20]. The most effective treatment for moderate and severe OSA is continuous positive airway pressure (CPAP) therapy, which stabilizes breathing throughout the night, improves daytime sleepiness and quality of life, and reduces risk of motor-vehicle accidents [15,19,21,22]. However, CPAP therapy requires patients to wear pressurized nasal/oro-nasal masks throughout the night, and is limited by poor patient acceptance and disappointing long-term adherence [23].

1.2. The Beginning of COMISA Research

Guilleminault, Eldridge, and Dement were the first to document the co-occurrence of insomnia and sleep apnea in 1973 [24]. Two middle-aged male patients were described, who presented with histories of chronic sleep maintenance and early morning awakening insomnia complaints. Both patients completed overnight polysomnography (PSG) studies at the Stanford Sleep Disorders Clinic, and were subsequently found to have significant sleep apnea. In 1976, Guilleminault and colleagues conducted a larger study to identify the proportion of chronic insomnia patients with occult OSA [25], and reported that of the 56 patients referred for symptoms of chronic insomnia, 10.7% were also found to have sleep apnea. Given that many insomnia patients are prescribed sedating benzodiazepine medications that can potentially exacerbate manifestations of OSA, Guilleminault and colleagues expressed substantial concern regarding the identification and management of COMISA patients [25]. Hence, this early COMISA research highlighted the importance of assessing insomnia patients for OSA symptoms, and recommended additional research to investigate the overlap of insomnia and OSA [24,25]. However, this prescient suggestion failed to attract research interest in the COMISA field for the subsequent three decades (Figure 1).

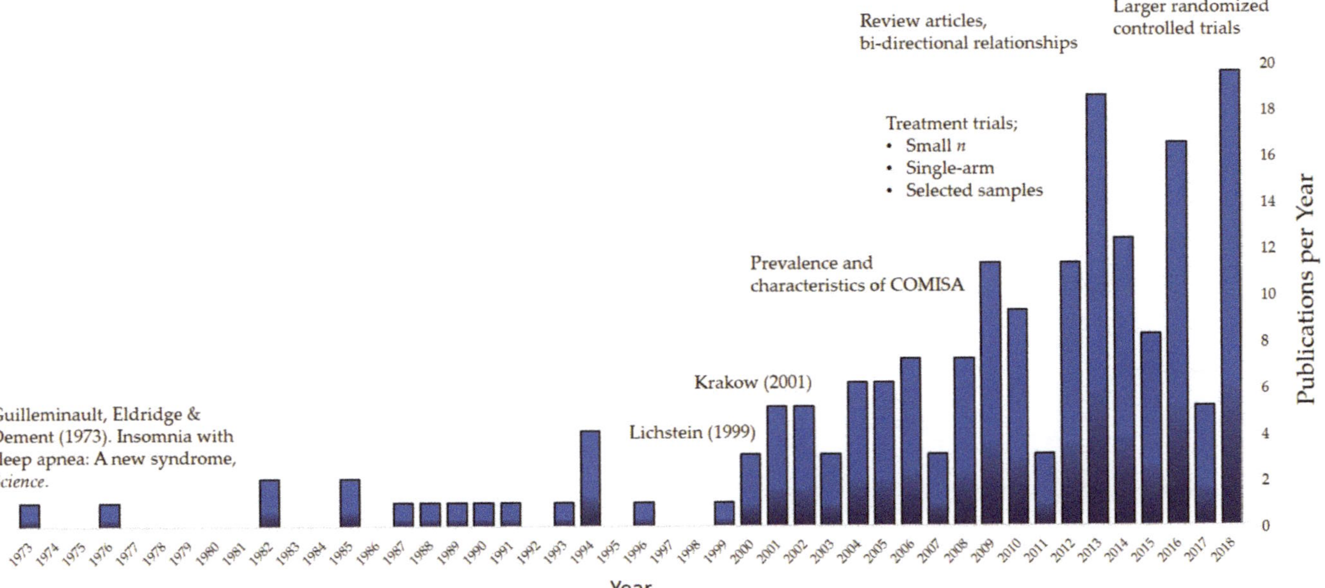

Figure 1. History of research in co-morbid insomnia and sleep apnea, including Guilleminault and colleague's 1973 article, and a lack of widespread research attention until two articles by Lichstein and colleagues (1999) and Krakow and colleagues (2001).

This lack of research attention possibly resulted from the differences in stereotypical characterizations of OSA and insomnia patient profiles, which mis-directed clinical attention, and research interest in their co-occurrence. For example, OSA has historically been conceptualized as a disorder impacting middle-aged and older-adult males, who are overweight or obese and present with complaints of excessive daytime sleepiness, tiredness, sedation, and snoring. Although epidemiological studies provide statistical support for these 'risk factors' (e.g., OSA is associated with male gender, increased age, overweight and obesity, snoring, and daytime sleepiness [14]), reliance on this single profile clearly does not represent all OSA sufferers [26–28]. Alternatively, insomnia has historically been conceptualized as a disorder primarily impacting middle-aged and older-adult females who are predisposed to anxiety, stress, and cycles of cognitive rumination. Although cross-sectional studies support the statistical association of these age, gender and personality characteristics with insomnia symptoms, this profile is not reflective of all insomnia sufferers [6]. Given that several risk factors and symptoms of OSA and insomnia occur in direct opposition (e.g., male vs. female sex, sleepiness vs. sleeplessness, sedation vs. anxiety), it seems counterintuitive that the two disorders should co-occur. Consequently, these historical conceptualizations of distinct insomnia- and OSA-profiles may have contributed to an attentional and referral bias against COMISA, which resulted in the 27 year period of research dormancy.

Alternatively, the lack of COMISA research following Guilleminault's 1973 publication may have also resulted from conceptualizations of 'primary' versus 'secondary' insomnia. Historically, when insomnia has co-occurred in the presence of another disorder, it has commonly been conceptualized as a 'secondary' condition, which is precipitated and maintained by the assumed 'primary' disorder [29]. This assumption implies that insomnia complaints will improve with successful treatment of the assumed 'primary' condition, and that the insomnia does not require independent diagnostic attention or targeted treatment [29–32]. Although insomnia is now recognized as an independent and self-perpetuating disorder which necessitates targeted diagnostic and therapeutic attention in the presence of co-occurring disorders [32,33], these historical mis-conceptualizations of 'secondary' insomnia may have also reduced research interest in COMISA during this period.

Although a handful of articles reported on the co-occurrence of insomnia and OSA following Guilleminault's seminal 1973 publication [34–36], widespread interest in COMISA was only re-ignited following two articles published in 1999 and 2001. In 1999, Lichstein and colleagues examined the incidence of OSA among 80 insomnia patients without obvious indicators of OSA (i.e., patients with symptoms indicative of OSA, including witnessed apneas, snoring, excessive daytime sleepiness, obesity, etc., were excluded from the study) [37]. Of the 80 insomnia patients, 43% had an AHI of at least five (indicative of at least mild OSA), and 29% had an AHI of at least 15 (indicative of at least moderate OSA) on an overnight PSG study. Alternatively, in 2001 Krakow and colleagues reported that among 231 OSA patients managed at a University Sleep Clinic 50% reported clinically significant insomnia symptoms, including at least two symptoms of either taking at least 30 min to fall asleep, waking up a lot, or having difficulty returning to sleep upon awakening [38]. Collectively, these two articles provided substantial evidence of the common co-morbidity of insomnia and OSA first reported by Guilleminault in 1973 [24], and provided a springboard for additional COMISA research. Figure 1 provides an overview of primary research, review articles, and conference abstracts in the COMISA research field per year, since Guilleminault's initial *Science* publication. In this narrative review, we plan to update and extend upon two previous reviews in the COMISA field [39,40], to describe the most recent and relevant research investigating the prevalence, consequences, methodological considerations, treatment approaches, and theoretical bi-directional relationships in COMISA. This recent research is integrated with previous literature to provide researchers and clinicians with clinical recommendations and future research directions.

1.3. COMISA Prevalence

The frequent co-occurrence of insomnia and OSA has since been confirmed by many research groups who have investigated a wide variety of samples and utilized a number of different tools and criteria to define insomnia, and OSA. In 2010 Luyster and colleagues reviewed COMISA literature, and concluded that 39%–58% of OSA patients report insomnia symptoms, and 29%–67% of insomnia patients fulfil minimal criteria for OSA [39]. In 2017, we subsequently published a review article in which we coined the term "COMISA", and reviewed prevalence estimates reported from 2010 to 2015, consequences, and early COMISA treatment research [40]. In our review of prevalence studies, we confirmed the high prevalence of COMISA, which varies considerably based on the initial disorder of interest (e.g., the prevalence of OSA in insomnia patients, or the prevalence of insomnia in OSA patients), the diagnostic tools and (severity) criteria for each disorder (e.g., requiring an AHI of five vs. 10 to diagnose OSA, or requiring formal diagnostic criteria for insomnia vs. self-reported symptoms via a brief questionnaire, etc.), and the population of interest (e.g., sleep clinic samples, general population, military personnel, etc.) [40]. Between 2013 and 2018, a number of large cluster analyses of OSA samples also identified that 32%–54% of OSA patients indicate symptoms of 'disturbed sleep', characterized by nocturnal insomnia symptoms, more frequent use of sedative-hypnotic medications, and lower use of CPAP therapy [26,27,41,42]. Most recently, Zhang and colleagues conducted a systematic review and meta-analysis including 37 studies investigating the co-morbidity of insomnia and OSA, and reported that 35% of insomnia patients have an AHI of ≥ 5, and 29% have an AHI of ≥ 15, while 38% of OSA patients meet insomnia criteria [43]. Interestingly, this meta-analysis excluded studies investigating veterans and samples comprised of trauma patients, in which even higher COMISA prevalence rates have been reported [44,45].

1.4. Consequences of COMISA

Importantly, COMISA patients experience greater impairments to daytime functioning and quality of life, compared to those with either insomnia, or OSA alone [40]. For example, Krakow and colleagues were among the first to report that compared to patients with OSA alone, COMISA patients expressed greater emotional and cognitive impairments, including irritability, reduced concentration, depressive symptoms, and anxiety [38]. In 2017, we reviewed a large number of studies which indicated an additive and substantial impairment to sleep, daytime functioning, depressive and psychiatric symptoms, and quality of life among COMISA patients [40]. Since 2017, a number of other studies have confirmed associations between COMISA and increased depressive and anxiety symptoms, daytime sleepiness, reduced quality of life, neurocognitive performance, and sleep quality compared to patients with either insomnia or OSA alone [46–52]. Hence, a large body of evidence has left little doubt that COMISA is a common disorder, which is associated with substantial impairments to nocturnal sleep, daytime functioning, and quality of life.

1.5. Refining the Measurement of COMISA

The presence and severity of insomnia has been defined according to a large range of measures and methods including structured and semi-structured interviews, self-report questionnaires, sleep diaries, and objective sleep recordings [53–57]. However, there has previously been a lack of research attention directed toward the validity of existing insomnia measures in the presence of OSA [58]. As insomnia and OSA share multiple overlapping symptoms, the diagnosis and measurement of each disorder in the presence of the other represents a complex task for researchers and clinicians [39,40,59].

Insomnia is diagnosed according to the frequency, severity, and chronicity of nocturnal sleep complaints and daytime impairments [1]. However, OSA commonly results in similar symptoms, including frequent post-apneic nocturnal awakenings, perceptions of nonrestorative sleep, daytime sleepiness and fatigue, and reduced quality of life [39,60]. It is possible that these shared symptoms result in an artefactual increase in the prevalence of COMISA, and complicate the assessment of changes in insomnia symptoms before and after different treatment approaches. For example, questionnaire measures of insomnia commonly include both nocturnal and daytime symptoms [54,55,61]. However, it is possible that many OSA patients may indicate elevated daytime impairments on these questionnaire measures in the absence of nocturnal insomnia complaints, resulting in higher overall 'insomnia' scores and a misclassification of COMISA. The same overlapping symptoms may also complicate the measurement of insomnia symptoms following different treatment approaches in COMISA. For example, COMISA patients treated with CPAP therapy may report a reduction of daytime impairments, which may translate to an overall reduction of 'insomnia severity' questionnaire scores in the absence of improved nocturnal symptoms.

To investigate the measurement of insomnia symptoms in the presence of OSA, Wallace and Wohlgemuth [62] recently examined profiles and predictors of insomnia severity index (ISI) questionnaire responses among 630 veterans with OSA. The ISI [54] is a brief, and valuable questionnaire measure of insomnia presence and severity, which has been utilized in several hundred insomnia treatment studies, including COMISA research [52,63–65]. The ISI includes seven self-report items, including three nocturnal items (difficulties falling asleep, staying sleep, and waking up too early), and four daytime items (satisfaction with sleep, daytime functioning interference, quality of life impairment, and worry/distress). These items are traditionally summed for a total score ranging from 0 to 28, with higher scores indicating more severe insomnia, and a score of ≥15 indicating clinically significant insomnia symptoms. Wallace and Wohlgemuth performed a latent profile analysis which identified that 30% of their OSA sample reported moderate insomnia, and an additional 44% reported severe insomnia. Importantly, these 'moderate' and 'severe' COMISA patients reported elevated nocturnal and daytime ISI symptoms. Wallace and Wohlgemuth propose that when administered to OSA patients, the ISI should be scored according to a 'nocturnal' sub-score (comprising the first three items, ranging from 0 to 12), and a 'daytime' sub-score (comprising the subsequent four items, ranging from 0 to 16). This 'nocturnal' score has also recently been investigated in other insomnia research [66,67], and has previously been utilized in several COMISA treatment studies [52,63,64].

It will be important for future research to validate different scoring criteria and cut-offs of the ISI and other insomnia questionnaire measures against psychologist-diagnostic criteria in the presence of OSA, to further refine the diagnosis and measurement of COMISA. Furthermore, future treatment research in COMISA samples should aim to include a range of outcomes measures which assess unique, and shared symptoms of each disorder.

2. Treatment of COMISA

2.1. Traditional Treatment Approaches

CPAP therapy is the most effective treatment for moderate and severe OSA [15,21]. Barthlen and colleagues were among the first to describe the association of insomnia symptoms and reduced CPAP adherence among two patients with severe OSA and insomnia symptoms [68]. Since this time, a large number of case studies [69], pilot studies [70,71], chart-reviews [65,72], treatment trials [44,49,50], and cluster analyses [41,42] have examined the effect of co-morbid insomnia symptoms on reduced CPAP outcomes in OSA patients. Although some studies report no association [63,73,74], the majority of research suggests that the presence of insomnia symptoms reduces CPAP acceptance and use. Understandably, patients who spend long periods awake wearing pressurized CPAP masks throughout the night, are more likely to experience CPAP-related side effects, and will be more likely to remove the CPAP equipment during the night, or reject CPAP therapy entirely.

This finding has led several groups to suggest that COMISA patients should be referred for insomnia treatment before commencing CPAP therapy. CBTi is the recommended 'first line' treatment for insomnia, and appears to be effective in the presence of co-morbid OSA [8,9,52]. Although several early pilot studies and a randomized controlled trial (RCT) reported mixed findings [69,75–77], more recent quasi-experimental and RCT data support the effectiveness of CBTi in COMISA patients [52,64,78,79]. For example, we previously reported a chart review of 455 insomnia patients treated with CBTi at an out-patient hospital insomnia treatment service, and found that there were no significant differences in insomnia improvements during treatment between the 141 patients with co-morbid OSA, and the 314 patients with insomnia alone [52]. Furthermore, there was no association between OSA severity (AHI) and changes in nocturnal insomnia symptoms during treatment, indicating that those without OSA and those with mild, moderate, and severe OSA experienced similar benefit from CBTi. Fung and colleagues, also recently compared the effectiveness of a five session CBTi intervention with a sleep-education control, among 134 adult veterans with insomnia alone (*n* = 39), and co-morbid insomnia and mild OSA (*n* = 95), and also found no differences in insomnia improvements during CBTi between patients with insomnia alone, and COMISA patients [78]. Finally, our recent RCT data from 145 COMISA patients with moderate and severe OSA, indicated that CBTi leads to greater improvement in ISI scores, diary-measured sleep parameters, and dysfunctional beliefs and attitudes about sleep by post-treatment, compared to a no-treatment control group [64].

Given the effect of co-morbid insomnia symptoms on reduced acceptance and use of CPAP therapy [40], it is also important to consider the effectiveness of non-CPAP therapies in the COMISA population. A small number of studies have investigated the effect of oral appliance devices, upper airway surgery, and nasal dilator strip therapy in the treatment of COMISA patients [75,80]. For example, Guilleminault and colleagues [77] reported that upper airway surgery significantly improved sleep parameters, sleep architecture, AHI, and daytime functioning in 30 patients with co-morbid insomnia and mild OSA. Alternatively, Krakow and colleagues reported that nasal dilator strip therapy improves insomnia symptoms and perceived sleep quality in patients with subjective symptoms indicative of sleep maintenance insomnia and OSA [81,82]. Future research should continue to examine the efficacy of these and other non-CPAP therapies among COMISA patients unable to tolerate CPAP therapy (e.g., oral appliance devices, positional devices, etc.).

2.2. Combined Treatments for COMISA

Krakow and colleagues were among the first to propose that COMISA patients have greater difficulties adapting to CPAP, and should be referred for CBTi before commencing CPAP therapy [38]. Two early studies provided preliminary support for the combination of CBTi and CPAP therapy in COMISA patients [76,83]. In 2001, Melendrez and colleagues reported a study examining the effect of CBTi followed by CPAP therapy in seven female crime victims with PTSD and COMISA [76]. They found that the patients experienced a significant six points ISI reduction following CBTi, and an additional six points ISI reduction following three subsequent months of CPAP therapy. Alternatively, Wickwire and colleagues reported a case study in which a middle-aged male with chronic insomnia and OSA was treated with a nine session CBTi program, which resulted in a small increase in CPAP use [83].

Until very recently, there have been very few trials examining the combination of CBTi and CPAP therapy in COMISA patients [39,40]. Table 1 displays an overview of recent RCTs investigating the combination of CBTi and CPAP therapy in COMISA. Bjorvatn and colleagues recently reported an RCT in which 134 COMISA patients were randomized to receive either a self-help CBTi book, or sleep hygiene information while commencing CPAP therapy [84]. The same research group previously found that the CBTi book resulted in significantly greater improvements in insomnia symptoms compared to sleep hygiene information material, among patients with insomnia alone [85]. In their recent COMISA study, although both the CBTi book and sleep hygiene control groups reported significant improvement of insomnia symptoms from pre- to post-treatment (change in ISI, and Bergen Insomnia Scale [86]), there was no difference in improvements between groups [84]. Similarly, there were also no differences in objective CPAP adherence over the first 3 months of treatment between groups (2.54 hours, versus 2.55 hours in the sleep hygiene and CBTi book groups, respectively). This lack of differences in insomnia and CPAP outcomes may be due to this sample reflecting patients primarily recruited for management of OSA, who were potentially less motivated to read and adhere to the instructions of the CBTi book. Indeed, 22% of the COMISA patients reported that they did not read the CBTi material, compared to only 5% of insomnia patients investigated in the previous RCT [84,85]. As the CBTi book and CPAP were commenced concurrently, it is also possible that patients derived sufficient benefit from CPAP alone, and did not perceive a need to utilize the CBTi intervention.

Table 1. Recent randomized controlled trials investigating the combination of CBTi and CPAP therapy for COMISA patients.

Study	n	Diagnostic Criteria	CBTi Intervention	Control	CPAP Follow-up	Insomnia Outcome	CPAP Use
Alessi et al., 2018 [79,87]	125	ICSD-3, AHI ≥ 15	Five session CBTi and behavioral CPAP adherence program, delivered concurrently with CPAP	Sleep Education Program	Objective CPAP data at 6 months.	CBTi group showed greater improvement during treatment.	CBTi group showed 78, and 48 min greater CPAP use, at the 3 and 6 month follow-ups, respectively.
Bjorvatn et al., 2018 [84]	134	DSM-5, ICSD-3, AHI ≥ 5	Previously validated self-help CBTi book, delivered concurrently with CPAP	Sleep hygiene advice	Objective CPAP data at 3 months.	No difference in improvement of ISI or Bergen Insomnia Scale between groups.	No significant difference between groups. Mean difference = 1 minute.
Ong et al., 2019 [88,89]	121	ICSD-2, AHI ≥ 5	Four session CBTi program, delivered before vs. concurrently with CPAP	No treatment, monitoring	Objective CPAP data at 3 months	CBTi groups reported greater ISI improvement during treatment.	No significant difference between CBTi and CPAP-only groups. CBTi before CPAP (M use = 148 min, SD = 137) CBTi with CPAP (M use = 152 min, SD = 155) CPAP only (M use = 181 min, SD = 155).
Sweetman et al., 2019 [64]	145	ICSD-3, AHI ≥ 15	Four session CBTi program delivered before CPAP	No treatment	Objective CPAP data at 6 months.	CBTi group reported greater improvement of the ISI, sleep diary parameters, and dysfunctional beliefs about sleep during treatment.	CBTi group showed 61 min greater CPAP use over the first 6 months. CBTi before CPAP (M use = 265, SD = 166) CPAP only (M use = 204, SD = 153).

AHI = Apnea/hypopnea index, CBTi = cognitive and behavioral therapy for insomnia, CPAP = continuous positive airway pressure therapy, DSM-5 = Diagnostic and statistical manual of mental disorders 5th ed, ICSD = International classification of sleep disorders, ISI = insomnia severity index, SD = standard deviation.

Alessi and colleagues recently reported the preliminary results of an RCT [79,87] comparing the effect of a five session combined CBTi and behavioral CPAP adherence program delivered by trained 'sleep coaches', versus a sleep education control program, on insomnia improvement and CPAP use by 6 month follow-up. The CBTi/adherence intervention was delivered concurrently with CPAP therapy (the first session was administered prior to commencing CPAP therapy, and the subsequent sessions were administered after commencing CPAP therapy). They recruited 125 adult veterans (96% male) with ICSD-3 insomnia, and an AHI of at least 15 (indicating moderate and severe OSA, however average AHI for the group was in the severe range; Mean AHI = 35). Compared to sleep education control, the CBTi group showed a greater improvement of diary- and actigraphy-measured sleep parameters, greater ISI reduction, and 78 and 48 min greater adherence to CPAP therapy at the 3 and 6 month follow-up, respectively.

Ong and colleagues also recently reported the preliminary results of an RCT [88,89] comparing the effects of three treatment approaches for COMISA on insomnia symptoms and CPAP adherence over the first 3 months. Intervention-arms included administering CBTi before commencing CPAP therapy, administering CBTi concurrently with CPAP therapy, and treating patients with CPAP therapy alone. Patients included 121 adults with ICSD-2 insomnia, and an AHI of at least five (although average AHI for the whole sample was 24, indicating moderate-to-severe OSA). There was a significant group by time interaction on ISI scores ($p < 0.001$), indicating that the two groups of patients receiving both CBTi and CPAP therapy showed a greater reduction of global insomnia severity during treatment, compared to patients receiving CPAP alone. Alternatively, there was no difference in ISI improvement between groups receiving initial, versus concurrent CBTi. There was no difference in CPAP adherence between any of the three groups by 3 months follow-up. Full results of this study are yet to emerge.

Finally, we recently reported an RCT comparing the effect of a four sessions individual/small group CBTi program, versus a no-treatment control group, on improvements in insomnia symptoms and subsequent acceptance and long-term objective use of CPAP therapy [64]. The manualized CBTi program was delivered by psychologists, and included sleep hygiene education, sleep restriction therapy, cognitive therapy, sleep misperception feedback, and relapse prevention. We recruited 145 patients with ICSD-3 insomnia, and an AHI of at least 15 (although average AHI for the sample was in the severe range; $M = 35$) from a Hospital Sleep Clinic, and an online advertising recruitment arm. Compared to the control group, we found that the CBTi group showed significantly greater improvement of sleep-diary parameters, the ISI, and dysfunctional sleep-related beliefs from pre- to post-CBTi, and subsequently showed greater initial acceptance of CPAP, and 61 min greater use by 6 months follow-up [64]. Like Alessi and colleagues [79], and Ong and colleagues [88], we also found that COMISA patients receiving both CBTi and CPAP therapy reported significantly greater improvement of global insomnia symptoms by 6 months follow-up.

2.3. Summary of Recent COMISA Randomized Controlled Trials

Together, these recent larger RCTs provide tentative support for the effect of therapist-administered CBTi in improving insomnia symptoms and increasing subsequent use of CPAP therapy in COMISA patients. Firstly, it appears that CBTi delivered by trained therapists may be more effective than self-administered (bibliotherapy) CBTi materials for COMISA patients. Although Bjorvatn previously found that a self-administered CBTi book resulted in significantly greater insomnia improvements compared to a sleep hygiene control group in patients with insomnia alone [85], their more recent study indicated that COMISA patients were less likely to read the CBTi material, and showed no differences in insomnia improvements or CPAP use compared to the control group [84]. Alternatively, the recent RCTs [64,79,88] and previous studies [52,78] investigating therapist-delivered CBTi, indicate that when delivered in a face-to-face setting, CBTi is an effective insomnia treatment in the presence of co-morbid OSA. An additional study is currently investigating the effect of self-administered online CBTi in the treatment of COMISA [90].

Secondly, the avenue of patient referral and recruitment may impact the effectiveness of different treatment approaches. As discussed by Bjorvatn [84], patients presenting with a 'chief complaint' of OSA may show reduced motivation to adhere to CBTi instructions, and will experience little additional benefit from initial treatment with CBTi. Alternatively, patients presenting for the diagnosis/treatment of insomnia may be more likely to engage with CBTi, and therefore experience a greater effect of CBTi on improved sleep and CPAP outcomes. Differences in sample populations, recruitment, presenting symptoms and motivation for different treatments may partially explain the differences between these RCTs. For example, while Bjorvatn [84] primarily recruited patients referred for suspicion of OSA and found no effect of a self-administered CBTi book, Ong and colleagues recruited patients from a combination of community advertisements, word of mouth, referrals from other physicians and healthcare providers, and a pool of previous research participants, and found that CBTi effectively improved insomnia symptoms [89]. Alternatively, the participants in our study [64] were recruited from both sleep clinic populations (comprised of patients seeking a diagnosis and treatment for OSA), and an online recruitment arm (comprised of patients self-referred with symptoms indicative of insomnia and/or OSA), and showed a positive response to CBTi. The full results and recruitment pathways of Alessi and colleagues' study are yet to be reported [79]. It will be important for future research to investigate the effectiveness of different combined and singular treatment approaches, between patients presenting with a 'chief complaint' of either insomnia, OSA, or both disorders.

Regarding the sequential, versus concurrent delivery of CBTi and CPAP therapy, more data are needed to confirm the results and differences between these current trials, and guide clinical recommendations. While we demonstrated that initial treatment with CBTi was effective in improving initial acceptance and use of CPAP therapy [64], Alessi and colleagues [79] reported that concurrent delivery of CBTi increased CPAP use, while Ong and colleagues [88] reported no difference between initial or concurrent CBTi administration on CPAP outcomes, and Bjorvatn and colleagues [84] reported no effect of the concurrent administration of a CBTi book on insomnia or CPAP outcomes. Hence, there are substantial differences between these recent RCTs regarding the most effective sequence of treatments for COMISA. Given that co-morbid insomnia symptoms reduce acceptance of CPAP therapy, and that initial CPAP acceptance and use predicts future CPAP use [44,91], our recommendation is that CBTi should be initiated before commencing CPAP therapy to improve insomnia symptoms, and provide the greatest opportunity for a positive initial experience with CPAP therapy to encourage and maintain greater long-term adherence. However, the severity of patients' insomnia and OSA, and patient preferences for CBTi versus CPAP therapy as the initial treatment should also guide decisions regarding the use and timing of CBTi and CPAP therapy [92]. More research is also needed to determine whether any baseline symptoms or profiles predict the success of different sequences of CBTi and CPAP therapy in COMISA [40].

Alessi and colleagues' study [79,87], and our study [64] also included between-group CPAP data at both 3 and 6 month follow-up. Interestingly, while Alessi and colleagues observed a small decrease in CPAP use between the CBTi and control group between 3 month (CBTi group showed 78 min greater adherence) and 6 month follow-up (CBTi group showed 48 min greater CPAP adherence), we observed a stable maintenance of improved CPAP use in the CBTi group between 3 months (57 min greater adherence) and 6 months (64 min greater adherence). This difference in the maintenance of average CPAP use between CBTi and control groups, in these two studies may have resulted from the different control conditions (i.e., Alessi utilized a sleep education control, while we used a no-treatment control), or differences between study samples (e.g., Alessi's sample primarily included male veterans, while we recruited non-veteran patients recruited through a Hospital Sleep Clinic). Despite these small differences in between-group CPAP use, both the CBTi and control groups in each study appeared to show a pattern of gradually declining CPAP use over time.

Finally, while the CBTi interventions administered by Ong [88,89], Bjorvatn [84], and our own study [64] included multi-faceted CBTi approaches to target insomnia, Alessi and colleagues' intervention included a combination of CBTi components and CPAP-adherence strategies to simultaneously improve insomnia and encourage greater CPAP outcomes [79,87]. We chose to administer isolated treatments for insomnia, and OSA to investigate the relative contribution of each intervention to symptoms of COMISA [64]. However, given the success of previous motivational interviewing [93] and educational strategies [94] in improving CPAP acceptance and use, this combined strategy may prove to be the most effective for COMISA patients treated in clinical settings. Furthermore, as sleep clinics are encouraged to offer educational support for OSA patients commencing CPAP therapy [15], it may be possible to include CBTi interventions within these existing education platforms, to simultaneously target both insomnia symptoms and improved CPAP use [79].

3. Bi-Directional Relationships in COMISA

The high co-morbidity of insomnia and OSA are suggestive of underlying mechanistic bi-directional relationships, whereby symptoms of each disorder may pre-dispose patients to the development, or exacerbate the severity of the other [95,96]. For example, sleep loss may exacerbate manifestations of OSA. Several pilot-studies have reported that a full night of sleep deprivation reduces upper-airway muscle tone in normal sleepers [97–99], and results in an increased AHI and reduced minimum oxygen saturation in patients with suspected and mild OSA [100–103]. Furthermore, some evidence suggests that consecutive nights of partial sleep deprivation increase the frequency of respiratory events in patients with mild and moderate OSA [104]. Hence, it is possible that multiple consecutive or intermittent nights of partial sleep loss experienced by patients with chronic insomnia may contribute to the development or exacerbation of OSA.

Alternatively, insomnia disorder may be associated with a reduced respiratory arousal threshold, which may predispose patients to prematurely awaken to respiratory events [16,105]. Indeed, insomnia has been conceptualized as a disorder of chronic 'hyperarousal', including elevated cognitive (ruminations, anxiety, etc.) and physiological arousal (increased heart rate, sympathetic nervous system activity, etc.), which may include a reduced respiratory arousal threshold [3,106]. A greater frequency of post-apneic arousals and sleep onset events may increase time in 'transitional' light sleep and delay a patient's progression into deep sleep which is associated with a reduced AHI [107]. Interestingly, Janssen and colleagues recently reported case study data from a 75 year old male in which a CPAP adherence data indicated an increased residual AHI during acute episodes of stress-induced insomnia symptoms [108]. Given the possible role of insomnia symptoms in the development and exacerbation of OSA, it will be important for future research to examine the impact of treating the insomnia, on changes in the onset, frequency, and duration of respiratory events in patients with COMISA [109,110].

Alternatively, OSA may contribute to the development or exacerbation of insomnia. OSA is associated with frequent post-apneic arousals and surges in sympathetic activity throughout the night, which may lead to full awakenings, and insomnia complaints. Mercer and colleagues [111] previously demonstrated that upon awakening throughout the night, insomnia patients commonly misperceive prior sleep as wakefulness. It is possible that among COMISA patients, post-apneic awakenings are also associated with sleep-state misperceptions, culminating in perceptions of prolonged time to fall asleep initially or prolonged awakenings during the night and thus an insomnia complaint. Indeed, previous research has reported a reduction in sleep maintenance insomnia complaints among COMISA patients who are able to tolerate CPAP therapy [63,112]. Although insomnia symptoms may be initially precipitated by post-apneic arousals in many patients, insomnia disorder quickly develops functional independence of the initial precipitating factors, and demands targeted treatment approaches (see discussion of 'secondary' versus 'co-morbid' insomnia, above) [4,33].

Although several research groups have discussed the potential bi-directional relationships between COMISA, there has been a lack of research attention in this important area [39,40,95,108]. It will be possible to use data from current RCTs to examine the independent effects of CBTi and CPAP therapy on changes in the 'downstream' severity and manifestations of each disorder. Furthermore, this may provide a platform to investigate predictors of which patients show the greatest response to insomnia and OSA treatments in isolation.

4. Recommendations for Clinicians

- The majority of sleep clinics around the world currently specialize in the diagnosis and treatment of OSA whist neglecting the measurement and treatment of insomnia. However, 30%–50% of OSA patients report co-morbid insomnia symptoms, which reduce acceptance and use of CPAP therapy.
- Co-morbid insomnia symptoms commonly reduce CPAP use and contribute to higher impairment of daytime functioning and quality of life. Therefore, the insomnia symptoms demand targeted diagnostic and treatment considerations, and should not be assumed to be a 'secondary' manifestation of the OSA.
- Clinicians should administer sleep diaries [53], or the insomnia severity index [54] which can be scored with adjusted COMISA cut-offs [62], to screen for insomnia symptoms in patients with suspected OSA.
- COMISA patients should be treated with both CBTi and CPAP therapy to improve insomnia symptoms, and increase CPAP acceptance and use.
- CBTi should be delivered by psychologists, or trained therapists, who can also provide motivational CPAP support.

5. Future Research Directions

- The diagnosis of co-morbid insomnia and OSA represents a complex task due to shared diagnostic symptoms. It is important to validate and refine insomnia measures in the presence of OSA.
- Investigate baseline symptoms and profiles which predict successful responses to different treatment combinations and sequences in COMISA.
- Investigate bi-directional relationships between COMISA, by examining 1) the effect of CBTi on manifestations and severity of OSA (e.g., AHI [109]), and 2) examine the effect of CPAP therapy on manifestations and severity of insomnia symptoms (e.g., sleep parameters, sleep misperceptions, ISI, etc.).
- Determine the most effective CBTi components and combinations to treat insomnia and improve CPAP adherence (for example, using isolated CBTi components such as bedtime restriction therapy to increase sleep efficiency before commencing CPAP therapy).
- Continue examining the efficacy of non-CPAP therapies in the presence of co-morbid insomnia symptoms, for patients who reject CPAP therapy.

6. Conclusions

Although COMISA was first identified by Guilleminault and colleagues in 1973, there was a lack of research attention until the publication of two papers in 1999 and 2001 indicating a 30%–50% co-morbid prevalence rate. Subsequent research indicated that COMISA patients experience greater impairment of sleep, daytime functioning, and quality of life, compared to patients with either insomnia, or OSA alone. However, despite these additive impairments, COMISA patients also show worse acceptance and use of CPAP therapy, compared to patients with OSA alone. A number of recent RCTs have provided evidence that CBTi is an effective insomnia treatment in the presence of co-morbid OSA. Furthermore, COMISA patients treated with CBTi show increased initial acceptance and long-term use of CPAP therapy, compared to treatment with CPAP alone. It is recommended that clinicians utilize simple instruments to detect insomnia symptoms in OSA patients, and refer identified COMISA patients for combined CBTi and CPAP therapy. It will be important for future research to examine mechanistic bi-directional relationships between COMISA, and continue to refine and tailor different treatment combinations and sequences.

Author Contributions: A.S. reviewed literature for this article; A.S., L.L., and C.B. each provided significant input to the preparation and drafting of this article.

Acknowledgments: The authors would like to thank Jason Ong and Cathy Alessi for providing information about the Methods and Results of their recent COMISA RCTs.

Conflicts of Interest: The authors declare no conflict of interest.

Abbreviations

AHI	Apnea/hypopnea index
CBTi	Cognitive and behavioral therapy for insomnia
COMISA	Co-morbid insomnia and sleep apnea
CPAP	Continuous positive airway pressure
ISI	Insomnia severity index
OSA	Obstructive sleep apnea
PSG	Polysomnography
RCT	Randomized controlled trial

References

1. The American Academy of Sleep Medicine. *International Classification of Sleep Disorders (ICSD-3), Diagnostic and Coding Manual*, 3rd ed.; The American Academy of Sleep Medicine: Westchester, IL, USA, 2014.
2. American Psychological Association. *Diagnostic and Statistical Manual of Mental Disorders (DSM-5)*; American Psychiatric Publishing: Washington, DC, USA, 2013.
3. Bonnet, M.H.; Arand, D.L. Hyperarousal and Insomnia: State of the Science. *Sleep Med. Rev.* **2010**, *14*, 9–15. [CrossRef]
4. Perlis, M.; Smith, M.T.; Pigeon, W.R. Etiology and pathophysiology of insomnia. In *Principles and Practice in Sleep Medicine*, 4th ed.; Kryger, M.H., Roth, T., Dement, W.C., Eds.; Elsevier: Philadelphia, PA, USA, 2005; pp. 714–725.
5. Spielman, A.J.; Caruso, L.S.; Glovinsky, P.B. A behavioral perspective on insomnia treatment. *Psychiatry Clin. N. Am.* **1987**, *10*, 541–553. [CrossRef]
6. Ohayon, M.M. Epidemiology of insomnia: What we know and what we still need to learn. *Sleep Med. Rev.* **2002**, *6*, 97–111. [CrossRef]
7. Ohayon, M.M.; Reynolds, C.F. Epidemiological and clinical relevance of insomnia diagnosis algorithms according to the DSM-IV and the International Classification of Sleep Disorders (ICSD). *Sleep Med.* **2009**, *10*, 952–960. [CrossRef]
8. Qaseem, A.; Kansagara, D.; Forciea, M.A.; Cooke, M.; Denberg, T.D. Management of chronic insomnia disorder in adults: A clinical practice guideline from the American College of Physicians. *Ann. Intern. Med.* **2016**, *165*, 125–133. [CrossRef]
9. Schutte-Rodin, S.; Broch, L.; Buysse, D.; Dorsey, C.; Sateia, M. Clinical guideline for the evaluation and management of chronic insomnia in adults. *J. Clin. Sleep Med.* **2008**, *4*, 487–504.
10. Ree, M.; Junge, M.; Cunnington, D. Australasian Sleep Association position statement regarding the use of psychological/behavioral treatments in the management of insomnia in adults. *Sleep Med.* **2017**, *36*, S43–S47. [CrossRef]
11. Wilson, S.; Anderson, K.; Baldwin, D.; Dijk, D.-J.; Espie, A.; Espie, C.; Gringras, P.; Krystal, A.; Nutt, D.; Selsick, H. British Association for Psychopharmacology consensus statement on evidence-based treatment of insomnia, parasomnias and circadian rhythm disorders: An update. *J. Psychopharmacol.* **2019**, *33*, 923–947. [CrossRef]
12. Miller, C.B.; Valenti, L.; Harrison, C.M.; Bartlett, D.J.; Glozier, N.; Cross, N.E.; Grunstein, R.R.; Britt, H.C.; Marshall, N.S. Time trends in the family physician management of insomnia: The Australian experience (2000–2015). *J. Clin. Sleep Med.* **2017**, *13*, 785–790. [CrossRef]
13. Kaufmann, C.N.; Spira, A.P.; Depp, C.A.; Mojtabai, R. Long-term use of benzodiazepines and nonbenzodiazepine hypnotics, 1999–2014. *Psychiatr. Serv.* **2017**, *69*, 235–238. [CrossRef]
14. Punjabi, N.M. The epidemiology of adult obstructive sleep apnea. *Proc. Am. Thor. Soc.* **2008**, *5*, 136–143. [CrossRef]

15. Epstein, L.J.; Kristo, D.; Strollo, P.J.; Friedman, N.; Malhotra, A.; Patil, S.P.; Ramar, K.; Rogers, R.; Schwab, R.J.; Weaver, E.M.; et al. Clinical guideline for the evaluation, management and long-term care of obstructive sleep apnea in adults: Adult obstructive sleep apnea task force of the American Academy of Sleep Medicine. *J. Clin. Sleep Med.* **2009**, *5*, 263–276.
16. Osman, A.M.; Carter, S.G.; Carberry, J.C.; Eckert, D.J. Obstructive sleep apnea: Current perspectives. *Nat. Sci. Sleep* **2018**, *10*, 21–34. [CrossRef]
17. Kapur, V.K.; Baldwin, C.M.; Resnick, H.E.; Gottlieb, D.J.; Nieto, F.J. Sleepiness in patients with moderate to severe sleep-disordered breathing. *Sleep* **2005**, *28*, 472–478. [CrossRef]
18. Sassani, A.; Findley, L.J.; Kryger, M.; Goldlust, E.; George, C.; Davidson, T.M. Reducing motor-vehicle collisions, costs, and fatalities by treating obstructive sleep apnea syndrome. *Sleep* **2004**, *27*, 453–458. [CrossRef]
19. Ellen, R.L.; Marshall, S.C.; Palayew, M.; Molnar, F.J.; Wilson, K.G.; Man-Son-Hing, M. Systematic review of motor vehicle crash risk in persons with sleep apnea. *J. Clin. Sleep Med.* **2006**, *2*, 193–200.
20. Peppard, P.E.; Young, T.; Barnet, J.H.; Palta, M.; Hagen, E.W.; Hla, K.M. Increased prevalence of sleep-disordered breathing in adults. *Am. J. Epidemiol.* **2013**, *177*, 1006–1014. [CrossRef]
21. Kushida, C.A.; Chediak, A.; Berry, R.B.; Brown, L.K.; Gozal, D.; Iber, C.; Parthasarathy, S.; Quan, S.F.; Rowley, J.A. Clinical guidelines for the manual titration of positive airway pressure in patients with obstructive sleep apnea. *J. Clin. Sleep Med.* **2008**, *4*, 157–171.
22. McEvoy, R.D.; Antic, N.A.; Heeley, E.; Luo, Y.; Ou, Q.; Zhang, X.; Mediano, O.; Chen, R.; Drager, L.F.; Liu, Z. CPAP for prevention of cardiovascular events in obstructive sleep apnea. *N. Engl. J. Med.* **2016**, *375*, 919–931. [CrossRef]
23. Weaver, T.E.; Grunstein, R.R. Adherence to continuous positive airway pressure therapy: The challenge to effective treatment. *Proc. Am. Thor. Soc.* **2008**, *5*, 173–178. [CrossRef]
24. Guilleminault, C.; Eldridge, F.L.; Dement, W.C. Insomnia with sleep apnea: A new syndrome. *Science* **1973**, *181*, 856–858. [CrossRef]
25. Guilleminault, C.; Eldridge, F.L.; Phillips, J.R.; Dement, W.C. Two occult causes of insomnia and their therapeutic problems. *Arch. Gen. Psychiatry* **1976**, *33*, 1241–1245. [CrossRef]
26. Saaresranta, T.; Hedner, J.; Bonsignore, M.R.; Riha, R.L.; McNicholas, W.T.; Penzel, T.; Antalainen, U.; Kvamme, J.A.; Pretl, M.; Sliwinski, P. Clinical phenotypes and comorbidity in European sleep apnoea patients. *PLoS ONE* **2016**, *11*, e0163439. [CrossRef]
27. Ye, L.; Pien, G.W.; Ratcliffe, S.J.; Björnsdottir, E.; Arnardottir, E.S.; Pack, A.I.; Benediktsdottir, B.; Gislason, T. The different clinical faces of obstructive sleep apnoea: A cluster analysis. *Eur. Res. J.* **2013**, *44*, 1600–1607. [CrossRef]
28. Appleton, S.; Gill, T.; Taylor, A.; McEvoy, D.; Shi, Z.; Hill, C.; Reynolds, A.; Adams, R. Influence of gender on associations of obstructive sleep apnea symptoms with chronic conditions and quality of life. *Int. J Environ. Res. Pub. Health* **2018**, *15*, 930. [CrossRef]
29. Lichstein, K.L. Secondary insomnia: A myth dismissed. *Sleep Med. Rev.* **2006**, *10*, 3–5. [CrossRef]
30. Lichstein, K.; McCrae, C.; Wilson, N. *Secondary insomnia: Diagnostic issues, cognitive-behavioral treatment, and future directions. Treating Sleep Disorders: Principles and Practice of Behavioral Sleep Medicine*; Wiley: Hoboken, NJ, USA, 2003; pp. 286–304.
31. Lichstein, K.L.; Nau, S.D.; McCrae, C.S.; Stone, K.C. Psychological and behavioral treatments for secondary insomnias. In *Principles and Practice in Sleep Medicine*, 4th ed.; Kryger, M.H., Roth, T., Dement, W.C., Eds.; Elsevier: Philadelphia, PA, USA, 2005.
32. Stepanski, E.; Rybarczyk, B. Emerging research on the treatment and etiology of secondary or comorbid insomnia. *Sleep Med. Rev.* **2006**, *10*, 7–18. [CrossRef]
33. National Institutes of Health. National Institutes of Health State of the Science Conference statement on Manifestations and Management of Chronic Insomnia in Adults, June 13–15, 2005. *Sleep* **2005**, *28*, 1049–1057. [CrossRef]
34. Morin, C.M.; Kowatch, R.A.; Barry, T.; Walton, E. Cognitive-behavior therapy for late-life insomnia. *J. Consult. Clin. Psychol.* **1993**, *61*, 137–146. [CrossRef]
35. Stone, J.; Morin, C.M.; Hart, R.P.; Remsberg, S.; Mercer, J. Neuropsychological functioning in older insomniacs with or without obstructive sleep apnea. *Psychol. Aging* **1994**, *9*, 231. [CrossRef]

36. Coleman, R.M.; Roffwarg, H.P.; Kennedy, S.J.; Guilleminault, C.; Cinque, J.; Cohn, M.A.; Karacan, I.; Kupfer, D.J.; Lemmi, H.; Miles, L.E.; et al. Sleep-wake disorders based on a polysomnographic diagnosis. A national cooperative study. *J. Am. Med. Assoc.* **1982**, *147*, 997–1003.

37. Lichstein, K.L.; Riedel, B.W.; Lester, K.W.; Aguillard, R.N. Occult sleep apnea in a recruited sample of older adults with insomnia. *J. Consult. Clin. Psychol.* **1999**, *67*, 405–410. [CrossRef]

38. Krakow, B.; Melendrez, D.; Ferreira, E.; Clark, J.; Warner, T.D.; Sisley, B.; Sklar, D. Prevalence of insomnia symptoms in patients with sleep-disordered breathing. *Chest* **2001**, *120*, 1923–1929. [CrossRef]

39. Luyster, F.S.; Buysse, D.J.; Strollo, P.J. Comorbid insomnia and obstructive sleep apnea: Challenges for clinical practice and research. *J. Clin. Sleep Med.* **2010**, *6*, 196–204.

40. Sweetman, A.; Lack, L.C.; Catcheside, P.G.; Antic, N.A.; Chai-Coetzer, C.L.; Smith, S.S.; Douglas, J.A.; McEvoy, R.D. Developing a successful treatment for co-morbid insomnia and sleep apnoea. *Sleep Med. Rev.* **2017**, *33*, 28–38. [CrossRef]

41. Gagnadoux, F.; Vaillant, M.L.; Paris, A.; Pigeanne, T.; Leclair-Visonneau, L.; Bizieux-Thaminy, A.; Alizon, C.; Humeau, M.P.; Nguyen, XL.; Rouault, B.; et al. Relationship between OSA clinical phenotypes and CPAP treatment outcomes. *Chest* **2016**, *149*, 288–290. [CrossRef]

42. Pien, G.W.; Ye, L.; Keenan, B.T.; Maislin, G.; Björnsdóttir, E.; Arnardottir, E.S.; Benediktsdottir, B.; Gislason, T.; Pack, A.I. Changing Faces of OSA: Treatment Effects by Cluster Designation in the Icelandic Sleep Apnea Cohort. *Sleep* **2018**, *41*, zsx201. [CrossRef]

43. Zhang, Y.; Ren, R.; Lei, F.; Zhou, J.; Zhang, J.; Wing, Y.-K.; Sanford, L.D.; Tang, X. Worldwide and regional prevalence rates of co-occurrence of insomnia and insomnia symptoms with obstructive sleep apnea: A systematic review and meta-analysis. *Sleep Med. Rev.* **2019**, *45*, 1–17. [CrossRef]

44. Wallace, D.M.; Vargas, S.S.; Schwartz, S.J.; Aloia, M.S.; Shafazand, S. Determinants of continuous positive airway pressure adherence in a sleep clinic cohort of South Florida Hispanic veterans. *Sleep Breath.* **2013**, *17*, 351–363. [CrossRef]

45. Mysliwiec, V.; Matsangas, P.; Baxter, T.; McGraw, L.; Bothwell, N.E.; Roth, B.J. Comorbid insomnia and obstructive sleep apnea in military personnel: Correlation with polysomnographic variables. *Mil. Med.* **2014**, *179*, 294–300. [CrossRef]

46. Lang, C.J.; Appleton, S.L.; Vakulin, A.; McEvoy, R.D.; Wittert, G.A.; Martin, S.A.; Catcheside, P.G.; Antic, N.A.; Lack, L.; Adams, R. Co-morbid OSA and insomnia increases depression prevalence and severity in men. *Respirology* **2017**, *22*, 1407–1415.

47. Tasbakan, M.; Gunduz, C.; Pirildar, S.; Basoglu, O.K. Quality of life in obstructive sleep apnea is related to female gender and comorbid insomnia. *Sleep Breath.* **2018**, *22*, 1013–1020. [CrossRef]

48. Cho, Y.; Kim, K.T.; Moon, H.J.; Korostyshevskiy, V.R.; Motamedi, G.K.; Yang, K.K. Comorbid Insomnia with Obstructive Sleep Apnea: Clinical Characteristics and Risk Factors. *J. Clin. Sleep Med.* **2018**, *14*, 409–417. [CrossRef]

49. Wallace, D.M.; Sawyer, A.; Shafazand, S. Comorbid insomnia symptoms predict lower 6-month adherence to CPAP in US veterans with obstructive sleep apnea. *Sleep Breath.* **2018**, *22*, 5–15. [CrossRef]

50. El-Solh, A.A.; Adamo, D.; Kufel, T. Comorbid insomnia and sleep apnea in Veterans with post-traumatic stress disorder. *Sleep Breath.* **2018**, *22*, 23–31. [CrossRef]

51. Philip, R.; Catcheside, P.; Stevens, D.; Lovato, N.; McEvoy, D.; Vakulin, A. Comorbid insomnia and sleep apnoea is associated with greater neurocognitive impairment compared with OSA alone. *J. Sleep Res.* **2017**, *40*, e260. [CrossRef]

52. Sweetman, A.; Lack, L.C.; Lambert, S.; Gradisar, M.; Harris, J. Does co-morbid obstructive sleep apnea impair the effectiveness of cognitive and behavioral therapy for insomnia? *Sleep Med.* **2017**, *39*, 38–46. [CrossRef]

53. Buysse, D.J.; Ancoli-Israel, S.; Edinger, J.D.; Lichstein, K.L.; Morin, C.M. Recommendations for a standard research assessment of insomnia. *Sleep* **2006**, *29*, 1155–1173. [CrossRef]

54. Bastien, C.H.; Vallières, A.; Morin, C.M. Validation of the insomnia severity index as an outcome measure for insomnia research. *Sleep Med.* **2001**, *2*, 297–307. [CrossRef]

55. Soldatos, C.R.; Dikeos, D.G.; Paparrigopoulos, T.J. Athens Insomnia Scale: Validation of an instrument based on ICD-10 criteria. *J. Psychosom. Res.* **2000**, *48*, 555–560. [CrossRef]

56. Partinen, M.; Gislason, T. Basic Nordic Sleep Questionnaire (BNSQ): A quantitated measure of subjective sleep complaints. *J. Sleep Res.* **1995**, *4*, 150–155. [CrossRef] [PubMed]

57. Buysse, D.J.; Reynolds III, C.F.; Monk, T.H.; Hoch, C.C.; Yeager, A.L.; Kupfer, D.J. Quantification of subjective sleep quality in healthy elderly men and women using the Pittsburgh Sleep Quality Index (PSQI). *Sleep* **1991**, *14*, 331–338. [PubMed]

58. Sweetman, A.; Lack, L.C.; McEvoy, D. Refining the Measurement of Insomnia in Patients with Obstructive Sleep Apnea: Commentary on Wallace and Wohlgemuth. Predictors of Insomnia Severity Index Profiles in US veterans with Obstructive Sleep Apnea. *J. Clin. Sleep Med.* **2019**, in press.

59. Duarte, R.; Magalhães-da-Silveira, J.F.; Oliveira-e-Sá, T.S.; Rabahi, M.F.; Mello, F.C.; Gozal, D. Predicting Obstructive Sleep Apnea in Patients with Insomnia: A Comparative Study with Four Screening Instruments. *Lung* **2019**, *197*, 451–458. [CrossRef] [PubMed]

60. Chervin, R.D. Sleepiness, fatigue, tiredness, and lack of energy in obstructive sleep apnea. *Chest* **2000**, *118*, 372–379. [CrossRef]

61. Espie, C.A.; Kyle, S.D.; Hames, P.; Gardani, M.; Fleming, L.; Cape, J. The Sleep Condition Indicator: A clinical screening tool to evaluate insomnia disorder. *BMJ Open* **2014**, *4*, e004183. [CrossRef]

62. Wallace, D.M.; Wohlgemuth, W.K. Predictors of Insomnia Severity Index Profiles in US Veterans with Obstructive Sleep Apnea. *J. Clin. Sleep Med.* **2019**, in press.

63. Glidewell, R.N.; Renn, B.N.; Roby, E.; Orr, W.C. Predictors and patterns of insomnia symptoms in OSA before and after PAP therapy. *Sleep Med.* **2014**, *15*, 899–905. [CrossRef]

64. Sweetman, A.; Lack, L.; Catcheside, P.; Antic, N.; Smith, S.; Chai-Coetzer, C.L.; Douglas, P.; O'Grady, A.; Dunn, N.; Robinson, J.; et al. Cognitive and behavioral therapy for insomnia increases the use of continuous positive airway pressure therapy in obstructive sleep apnea participants with co-morbid insomnia: A randomized clinical trial. *Sleep* **2019**. [CrossRef]

65. Philip, P.; Bioulac, S.; Altena, E.; Morin, C.M.; Ghorayeb, I.; Coste, O.; Monteyrol, P.J.; Micoulaud-Franchi, JA. Specific insomnia symptoms and self-efficacy explain CPAP compliance in a sample of OSAS patients. *PLoS ONE* **2018**, *13*, e0195343. [CrossRef]

66. Ji, X.B.C.; Ellis, J.G.; Hale, L.; Grandner, M.A. Disassembling insomnia symptoms and their associations with depressive symptoms in a community sample: The differential role of sleep symptoms, daytime symptoms, and perception symptoms of insomnia. *Sleep Health* **2019**, *5*, 376–381. [CrossRef] [PubMed]

67. Otte, J.L.; Bakoyannis, G.; Rand, K.L.; Ensrud, K.E.; Guthrie, K.A.; Joffe, H.; McCurry, S.M.; Newton, K.M.; Carpenter, J.S. Confirmatory factor analysis of the Insomnia Severity Index (ISI) and invariance across race: A pooled analysis of MsFLASH data. *Menopause* **2019**, *26*, 850–855. [CrossRef] [PubMed]

68. Barthlen, G.M.; Lange, D.J. Unexpectedly severe sleep and respiratory pathology in patients with amyotrophic lateral sclerosis. *Eur. J. Neurol.* **2000**, *7*, 299–302. [CrossRef] [PubMed]

69. An, H.; Chung, S. A case of obstructive sleep apnea syndrome presenting as paradoxical insomnia. *Psychiatry Investig.* **2010**, *7*, 75–78. [CrossRef]

70. Smith, S.S.; Dunn, N.; Douglas, J.; Jorgensen, G. Sleep onset insomnia is associated with reduced adherence to CPAP therapy. *Sleep Biol. Rhythm.* **2009**, *7*, 74.

71. Suraiya, S.; Lavie, P. Sleep onset insomnia in sleep apnea patients: Influence on acceptance of nCPAP treatment. *Sleep Med.* **2006**, *7*, S85. [CrossRef]

72. Wickwire, E.M.; Smith, M.T.; Birnbaum, S.; Collop, N.A. Sleep maintenance insomnia complaints predict poor CPAP adherence: A clinical case series. *Sleep Med.* **2010**, *11*, 772–776. [CrossRef]

73. Nguyên, X.; Chaskalovic, J.; Rakotonanahary, D.; Fleury, B. Insomnia symptoms and CPAP compliance in OSAS patients: A descriptive study using data mining methods. *Sleep Med.* **2010**, *11*, 777–784. [CrossRef]

74. Mysliwiec, V.; Capaldi, V.; Gill, J.; Baxter, T.; O'Reilly, B.M.; Matsangas, P.; Roth, B.J. Adherence to positive airway pressure therapy in U.S. military personnel with sleep apnea improves sleepiness, sleep quality, and depressive symptoms. *Mil. Med.* **2015**, *180*, 475–482. [CrossRef]

75. Guilleminault, C.; Palombini, L.; Poyares, D.; Chowdhuri, S. Chronic insomnia, premenopausal women, and sleep disordered breathing part 2. Comparison of nondrug treatment trials in normal breathing and UARS post menopausal women complaining of chronic insomnia. *J. Psychosom. Res.* **2002**, *53*, 617–623. [CrossRef]

76. Melendrez, D.C.; Krakow, B.J.; Johnston, L.; Sisley, B.; Warner, T.D. A prospective study on the treatment of complex insomnia—Insomnia plus sleep disordered breathing—In a small series of crime victims with PTSD. *Sleep* **2001**, *24*, A120.

77. Guilleminault, C.; Davis, K.; Huynh, N.T. Prospective randomized study of patients with insomnia and mild sleep disordered breathing. *Sleep* **2008**, *31*, 1527–1533. [CrossRef] [PubMed]

78. Fung, C.H.; Martin, J.L.; Josephson, K.; Fiorentino, L.; Dzierzewski, J.M.; Jouldjian, S.; Rodriguez-Tapia, J.C.; Mitchell, M.N.; Alessi, C. Efficacy of cognitive behavioral therapy for insomnia in older adults with occult sleep-disordered breathing. *Psychosom. Med.* **2016**, *78*, 629. [CrossRef] [PubMed]

79. Alessi, C.; Martin, J.; Fung, C.; Dzierzewski, J.; Fiorentino, L.; Stepnowsky, C.; Song, Y.; Rodriguez, R.C.; Zeidler, M.; Mitchell, M. 0407 Randomized Controlled Trial of an Integrated Behavioral Treatment in Veterans with Obstructive Sleep Apnea and Coexisting Insomnia. *Sleep* **2018**, *41* (Suppl. 1), A155. [CrossRef]

80. Machado, M.A.C.; de Carvalho, L.B.C.; Juliano, M.L.; Taga, M.; do Prado, L.B.F.; do Prado, G.F. Clinical co-morbidities in obstructive sleep apnea syndrome treated with mandibular repositioning appliance. *Respir. Med.* **2005**, *100*, 988–995.

81. Krakow, B.; Melendrez, D.; Sisley, B.; Warner, T.D.; Krakow, J. Nasal dilator strip therapy for chronic sleep maintenance insomnia: A case series. *Sleep Breath.* **2004**, *8*, 133–140. [CrossRef]

82. Krakow, B.; Melendrez, D.; Sisley, B.; Warner, T.D.; Krakow, J.; Leahigh, L.; Lee, S. Nasal dilator strip therapy for chronic sleep-maintenance insomnia and symptoms of sleep-disordered breathing: A randomized controlled trial. *Sleep Breath.* **2006**, *10*, 16–28. [CrossRef]

83. Wickwire, E.M.; Schumacher, J.A.; Richert, A.C.; Baran, A.S.; Roffwarg, H.P. Combined insomnia and poor CPAP compliance: A case study and discussion. *Clin. Case Stud.* **2008**, *7*, 267–286. [CrossRef]

84. Bjorvatn, B.; Berge, T.; Lehmann, S.; Pallesen, S.; Saxvig, IW. No Effect of a Self-help Book for Insomnia in Patients with Obstructive Sleep Apnea and Comorbid Chronic Insomnia—A Randomized Controlled Trial. *Front. Psychol.* **2018**, *9*, 2413. [CrossRef]

85. Bjorvatn, B.; Fiske, E.; Pallesen, S. A self-help book is better than sleep hygiene advice for insomnia: A randomized controlled comparative study. *Scand. J. Psychol.* **2011**, *52*, 580–585. [CrossRef]

86. Pallesen, S.; Bjorvatn, B.; Nordhus, I.H.; Sivertsen, B.; Hjornevik, M.; Morin, C.M. A new scale for measuring insomnia: The Bergen Insomnia Scale. *Percept. Mot. Ski.* **2008**, *107*, 691–706. [CrossRef]

87. Alessi, C. Novel Treatment of Comorbid Insomnia and Sleep Apnea in Older Veterans. 2014. Available online: https://clinicaltrials.gov/ct2/show/NCT02027558 (accessed on 1 October 2019).

88. Ong, J.C.; Crawford, M.R.; Wyatt, J.K.; Fogg, L.F.; Turner, A.D.; Dawson, S.C.; Edinger, J.D.; Kushida, C.A.; Abbott, S.M.; Malkani, R.G. 0379 A Randomized Controlled Trial Of CBT-I and CPAP For Comorbid Insomnia and OSA: Initial Findings from the MATRICS Study. *Sleep* **2019**, *42* (Suppl. 1), A154. [CrossRef]

89. Crawford, M.R.; Turner, A.D.; Wyatt, J.K.; Fogg, L.F.; Ong, J.C. Evaluating the treatment of obstructive sleep apnea comorbid with insomnia disorder using an incomplete factorial design. *Contemp. Clin. Trials* **2016**, *47*, 146–152. [CrossRef] [PubMed]

90. Edinger, J.; Manber, R. *Stepped-Care Management of Insomnia Co-Occurring with Sleep Apnea*; National Institute of Health: Denver, CO, USA, 2016.

91. Van Ryswyk, E.; Anderson, C.S.; Antic, N.A.; Barbe, F.; Bittencourt, L.; Freed, R.; Heeley, E.; Liu, Z.; Loffler, K.; Lorenzio-Filho, G.; et al. Predictors of long-term adherence to continuous positive airway pressure in patients with obstructive sleep apnea and cardiovascular disease. *Sleep* **2019**, *36*, 1929–1937. [CrossRef] [PubMed]

92. Ong, J.C.; Crawford, M.R.; Kong, A.; Park, M.; Cvengros, J.A.; Crisostomo, M.I.; Alexander, E.I.; Whatt, J.K. Management of obstructive sleep apnea and comorbid insomnia: A mixed-methods evaluation. *Behav. Sleep Med.* **2016**, *15*, 180–197.

93. Olsen, S.L.; Smith, S.S.; Oei, T.; Douglas, J. Motivational interviewing (MINT) improves continuous positive airway pressure (CPAP) acceptance and adherence: A randomised controlled trial. *J. Consult. Clin. Psychol.* **2012**, *80*, 151–163. [CrossRef]

94. Wozniak, D.; Lasserson, T.J.; Smith, I. Educational, supportive and behavioural interventions to improve usage of continuous positive airway pressure machines in adults with obstructive sleep apnoea. *Cochrane Database Syst. Rev.* **2014**, *1*. [CrossRef]

95. Benetó, A.; Gomez-Siurana, E.; Rubio-Sanchez, P. Comorbidity between sleep apnea and insomnia. *Sleep Med. Rev.* **2009**, *13*, 287–293. [CrossRef]

96. Lack, L.; Sweetman, A. Diagnosis and treatment of insomnia comorbid with obstructive sleep apnea. *Sleep Med. Clin.* **2016**, *11*, 379–388. [CrossRef]

97. Eckert, D.J.; Parikh, S.; White, D.P.; Jordan, A.S.; Merchia, P.; Malhotra, A. Sleep deprivation impairs genioglossus muscle responsiveness. *Am. J. Respir. Crit. Care Med.* **2011**, *183*, A6163.

98. Parikh, S.; White, D.; Jordan, A.; Merchia, P.; Malhotra, A.; Eckert, D. 36 Hours of Sleep Deprivation Reduces Genioglossus Muscle Activity during Hypercapnia and Inspiratory Resistive Loads during Wakefulness. *Sleep* **2011**, *34*, A153.

99. Leiter, J.C.; Knuth, S.L.; Bartlett, D. The effect of sleep deprivation on activity of the genioglossus muscle. *Am. Rev. Res. Dies.* **1985**, *132*, 1242–1245.

100. Persson, H.E.; Svanborg, E. Sleep deprivation worsens obstructive sleep apnea: Comparison between diurnal and nocturnal polysomnography. *Chest* **1996**, *109*, 645–650. [CrossRef] [PubMed]

101. Desai, A.V.; Marks, G.; Grunstein, R. Does sleep deprivation worsen mild obstructive sleep apnea? *Sleep* **2003**, *26*, 1038–1041. [CrossRef] [PubMed]

102. Guilleminault, C.; Rosekind, M. The arousal threshold: Sleep deprivation, sleep fragmentation, and obstructive sleep apnea syndrome. *Bull. Eur. Physiopathol. Respir.* **1981**, *17*, 341–349.

103. Guilleminault, C.; Silvestri, R.; Mondini, S.; Coburn, S. Aging and sleep apnea: Action of benzodiazepine, acetazolamide, alcohol, and sleep deprivation in a healthy elderly group. *J. Gerontol.* **1984**, *39*, 655–661. [CrossRef]

104. Stoohs, R.A.; Dement, W.C. Snoring and sleep-related breathing abnormality during partial sleep deprivation. *N. Engl. J. Med.* **1993**, *328*, 1279. [CrossRef]

105. Younes, M. Role of arousals in the pathogenesis of obstructive sleep apnea. *Am. J. Crit. Care Med.* **2004**, *169*, 623–633. [CrossRef]

106. Bonnet, M.H.; Arand, D.L. Hyperarousal and insomnia. *Sleep Med. Rev.* **1997**, *1*, 97–108. [CrossRef]

107. Ratnavadivel, R.; Chau, N.; Stadler, D.; Yeo, A.; McEvoy, D.R.; Catcheside, P.G. Marked reduction in obstructive sleep apnea severity in slow wave sleep. *J. Clin. Sleep Med.* **2009**, *5*, 519–524.

108. Janssen, H.C.; Venekamp, L.N.; Peeters, G.A.; Pijpers, A.; Pevernagie, D.A. Management of insomnia in sleep disordered breathing. *Eur. Res. Rev.* **2019**, *28*, 190080. [CrossRef]

109. Sweetman, A.; Lack, L.; Catcheside, P.; Antic, N.; Smith, S.; Chai-Coetzer, C.L.; Douglas, P.; O'Grady, A.; Dunn, N.; Robinson, J.; et al. *The Effect of Cognitive and Behavioural Therapy for Insomnia on Changes in Sleep Architecture and AHI in Patients with Co-Occurring Insomnia and Sleep Apnea*; World Sleep: Vancouver, BC, Canada, 2019; Available online: https://www.researchgate.net/publication/334506579_The_effect_of_cognitive_and_behavioural_therapy_for_insomnia_on_changes_in_sleep_architecture_and_AHI_in_patients_with_co-occurring_insomnia_and_sleep_apnea (accessed on 1 October 2019).

110. Sériès, F. Can improving sleep influence sleep-disordered breathing? *Drugs* **2009**, *69* (Suppl. 2), 77–91. [CrossRef]

111. Mercer, J.D.; Bootzin, R.R.; Lack, L. Insomniacs' perception of wake instead of sleep. *Sleep* **2002**, *25*, 559–566. [CrossRef]

112. Björnsdóttir, E.; Janson, C.; Sigurdsson, J.F.; Gehrman, P.; Perlis, M.; Juliusson, S.; Arnardottir, E.S.; Kuna, S.T.; Pack, A.I.; Gislason, T. Symptoms of insomnia among patients with obstructive sleep apnea before and after two years of positive airway pressure treatment. *Sleep* **2013**, *36*, 1901–1909. [CrossRef]

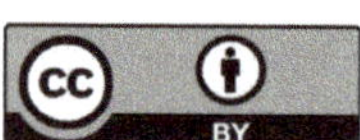

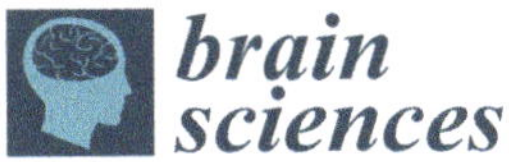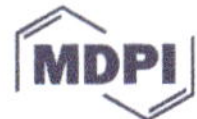

Article

Insomnia Might Influence the Thickness of Choroid, Retinal Nerve Fiber and Inner Plexiform Layer

Cigdem Sahbaz [1,*], Ahmet Elbay [2], Mine Ozcelik [3] and Hakan Ozdemir [2]

[1]   Department of Psychiatry, Faculty of Medicine, Bezmialem Vakıf University, Istanbul 34093, Turkey
[2]   Department of Ophthalmology, Bezmialem Vakıf University, Istanbul 34093, Turkey;
       draelbay@yahoo.com (A.E.); hozdemir72@hotmail.com (H.O.)
[3]   School of Medicine, Bezmialem Vakıf University, Istanbul 34093, Turkey; aysemineozcelik@gmail.com
*   Correspondence: cigdemdileksahbaz@gmail.com

Received: 13 February 2020; Accepted: 17 March 2020; Published: 19 March 2020

Abstract: Sleep may play a fundamental role in retinal regulation and the degree of retinal variables. However, no clinical study has investigated optical coherence tomography (OCT) parameters in patients with primary insomnia. All participants were evaluated with the insomnia severity index (ISI) and the Pittsburgh sleep quality index (PSQI). The retinal nerve fiber layer (RNFL), ganglion cell layer (GC), inner plexiform layer (IPL), macula and choroidal (CH) thickness were compared between 52 drug-naïve patients with primary insomnia and 45 age-gender-BMI-smoke status matched healthy controls (HC). The patients with primary insomnia differed from the HC regarding RNFL-Global ($p = 0.024$) and RNFL-Nasal inferior ($p = 0.010$); IPL-Temporal ($p < 0.001$), IPL-Nasal ($p < 0.001$); CH-Global ($p < 0.001$), CH-Temporal ($p = 0.004$), CH-Nasal ($p < 0.001$), and CH-Fovea ($p = 0.019$). ISI correlated with RNFL-Global and RNFL-Nasal inferior. The regression analysis revealed that ISI was the significant predictor for the thickness of RNFL- Nasal inferior ($p = 0.020$), RNFL-Global ($p = 0.031$), and CH-Nasal ($p = 0.035$) in patients with primary insomnia. Sleep disorders are seen commonly in patients with psychiatric, including ocular diseases. Adjusting the effect of insomnia can help to clarify the consistency in findings of OCT.

Keywords: OCT; insomnia disorder; sleep; retinal nerve fiber layer; choroid; inner plexiform layer

1. Introduction

Insomnia, persistent difficulty in initiating or maintaining sleep and corresponding daytime dysfunction, is a major public health issue and a common disorder associated with adverse long-term medical and psychiatric outcomes [1]. The prevalence of insomnia in the general population ranges between 8–40%, while the 20–30% of the general population has poor sleep [2], and the underlying pathophysiological mechanisms and causal relationships of insomnia with diseases are poorly understood [3]. The retina is a part of the central nervous system (CNS) and perceived as a "window to the brain" [4] in establishing similarities in the physiology and function of the CNS [5]. The retina also contains a circadian rhythm, and several studies have identified that many aspects of retinal physiology and functions are under the control of a retinal circadian system [6–8].

The release of the two primary neurotransmitters, dopamine (DA) and melatonin (MLT), provide the "day" and "night" signals in the retina, which reconfigure retinal circuits and shape the functioning of the retina according to the time of the day [6,9]. Dysfunction of the circadian rhythm within the retina affects adversely the retinal function in the processing of the light information, synaptic communication, and metabolism [8]. Taken together, sleep disturbances might have a role in retinal regulation and the grade of retinal variables.

Optic coherence tomography (OCT) provides a promising non-invasive and feasible methodological approach for investigating abnormalities in systemic conditions where possibly the degenerative changes are related to the optic nerve and retinal architecture [10]. Initial applications of OCT were limited mainly to ophthalmic diseases, but several studies found that the changes of the neural layers of the retina might predict CNS pathology such as cortical atrophy with patients in many non-ocular diseases [11,12]. Similarly, several studies on OCT tested the progression of the psychiatric disorders and found the thinning of RNFL or macula in patients with schizophrenia (SZ) [13], bipolar disorder (BP) [14], major depression (MD) [15], and anorexia nervosa [16]. However, the retinal findings were not strongly correlated with clinical symptoms in major psychiatric diseases [10]. Hence, the researchers suggested that the lack of consideration of potential confounder factors might explain the observed heterogeneity of the results of OCT parameters such as having metabolic diseases and using psychiatric medications [13].

According to our hypothesis, insomnia might be a potential confounder factor for the OCT findings in patients with major psychiatric disorders. A growing body of evidence demonstrates that sleep and circadian rhythm disruptions are associated with the pathophysiology of psychiatric [17] and neurodegenerative disorders [18,19]. Recent Genome-wide association analysis identified 57 loci associated with insomnia symptoms and asserted the evidence of shared genetic factors between insomnia and cardio-metabolic, behavioral, psychiatric, and reproductive traits [20]. Even more, studies among patients with ocular diseases such as blindness, glaucoma [21], and central serous chorioretinopathy (CSCR) [22] have reported a higher prevalence of sleep disturbances. Evidence supporting this hypothesis is coming from studies in which the obstructive sleep apnea syndrome (OSAS) recognized and treated showed that better anatomical and functional visual outcomes in patients with CSCR [23] and age-related macular degeneration [24] found after treatment. OSAS is a chronic respiratory-related sleep disorder and recognized as a risk factor for many systemic disorders, including hypertension, cardiovascular disease [23]. The respiratory component of OSAS may produce significant hypoxic tissue responses; however, it has not been investigated whether the retinal changes are caused by sleep component or respiratory component [25].

To the best of our knowledge, there is no study conducted to investigate the direct effect of sleep disorder such as primary insomnia on the retinal findings excluding the potential confounders. Therefore, we aim to explore the OCT parameters in fifty-two drug-naïve patients with primary insomnia compared with age-BMI-gender-smoking matched healthy controls. All participants were excluded from potential confounders such as relating primarily to ocular disorders, neuropsychiatric disorders, metabolic diseases, and drug use.

2. Materials and Methods

The sample consisted of 52 participants with primary insomnia, and 45 healthy control subjects, aged between 18 and 65 old. All participants were recruited from the psychiatry and ophthalmology outpatient clinics of a university hospital, i.e., Bezmialem Vakif University (Istanbul, Turkey). All participants were interviewed by senior psychiatrists. The primary insomnia was diagnosed based on DSM-IV (APA, 2000) criteria which consist of the predominant insomnia complaint with the difficulties on initiating and maintaining sleep with subjectively experienced daytime impairments, excluding any organic origin for at least 1-month period, additionally only the patients with primary insomnia considered eligible to take part in the study.

The healthy control subjects were recruited from a pool of the administrative staff of the hospital. Participants with mental retardation, psychotic disorders, mood disorders, obsessive compulsive disorder, substance use and dependence were excluded. Other exclusion criteria were as follows: (i) Any medical diagnoses, e.g. diabetes mellitus, hypertension, and metabolic syndrome, OSAS, (ii) neurodegenerative diseases, (iii) pathologies of the eye, anterior and posterior segment diseases including a history of ocular contusion, cataracts, glaucoma, corneal diseases, uveitis, macular degeneration, diabetic retinopathy, retinal diseases, amblyopia, neurologic disorders such as optic neuritis; also patients who had any previous ocular operation or trauma history were excluded.

The Medical Ethical Review Committee of the Bezmialem Vakif University approved the study (Date: 01.08.2017, Number 13/204) which was conducted according to the latest version of the Declaration of Helsinki. Written informed consent was obtained from all participants.

2.1. Procedure

All participants underwent a comprehensive ophthalmic examination, including corrected visual acuity measurement (with Snellen chart), slit-lamp biomicroscopy, intraocular pressure measurement and indirect ophthalmoscopy. Patients who had a spherical refractive error < −2 D or > +2 D and a visual acuity less than 1.0 were excluded from the study. All participants underwent OCT measurements including IPL, GCL, and choroidal thickness and peripapillary RNFL by the same experienced operator at the same time of the day (08:00 am–10:00 am). OCT measurements were performed without pupil dilation by using a Spectralis OCT device (software version 6.9, Heidelberg Engineering, Heidelberg, Germany). For peripapillary retinal nerve fiber layer (RNFL) thickness measurement, circular scans of 3.4 mm diameter centered on the optic disc were acquired. The images were automatically segmented into seven segments using the Heidelberg Eye Explorer software (version 1.9.10.0; Heidelberg Engineering) (Figure 1).

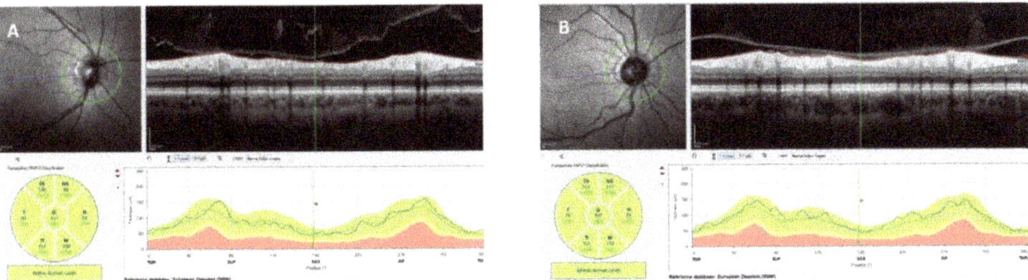

Figure 1. Peripapillary retinal nerve fiber layer (RNFL) thickness measurement. (**A**). A patient with primary insomnia. (**B**). A healthy individual. Top-left image: Scanning laser ophthalmoscopy image of the optic nerve. Green circle shows the corresponding OCT- circle scan shown in top-right image. Bottom-left image: Thickness map of the peripapillary RNFL thickness. While the inner 1-mm circle was defined as global RNFL peripapillary six area defined as temporal superior, temporal, temporal inferior, nasal inferior, nasal and nasal superior. Global RNFL was the mean value of these six regions.

To evaluate the GCL and IPL thickness measurement the horizontal scan crossing through the fovea was taken as a screening line. GHT and IPT thicknesses were measured from nasal and temporal points at a distance of 1000 μm to the fovea. Measurements were made by using the magnification option in the device software to enlarge four-fold the original image. As the GCL, the relative hyperreflective area between the bottom edge of the RNFL, which is the most hyperreflective band on the surface of the retina, and the upper edge of the hyporeflective area, the IPT, was accepted. The area between the bottom edge of GHT and the upper edge of the inner nuclear layer, which is a relatively hyperreflective area, was defined as IPT. To evaluate the choroidal thickness, OCT scans were acquired through the fovea with the horizontal 30-line-scan enhanced depth imaging mode of the device. The images were averaged over 100 scans using an automatic real-time imaging value of 100 and active eye-tracking features. Choroidal thickness measurements were made manually at the central fovea and at 1000 μm nasal and temporal points to the fovea. The mean value of these three measures was accepted as the choroidal thickness. The manual callipers and 2× magnification option provided with the device software were used. The distance between the outer part of the hyperreflective line corresponding to RPE-BM and the hyporeflective line corresponding to the choroid-scleral junction was evaluated as choroidal thickness (Figure 2).

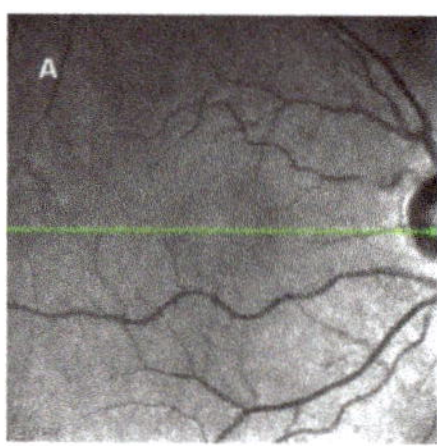 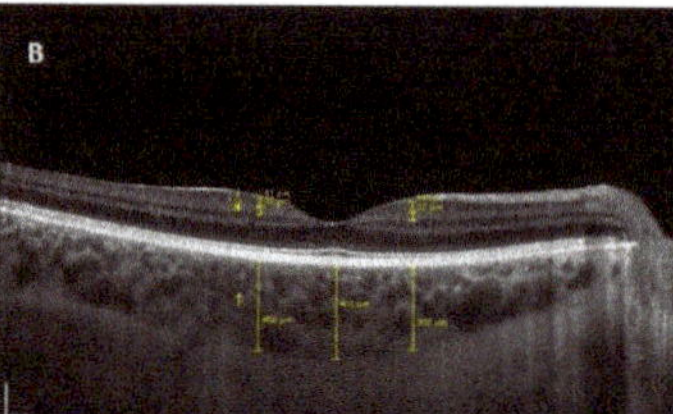 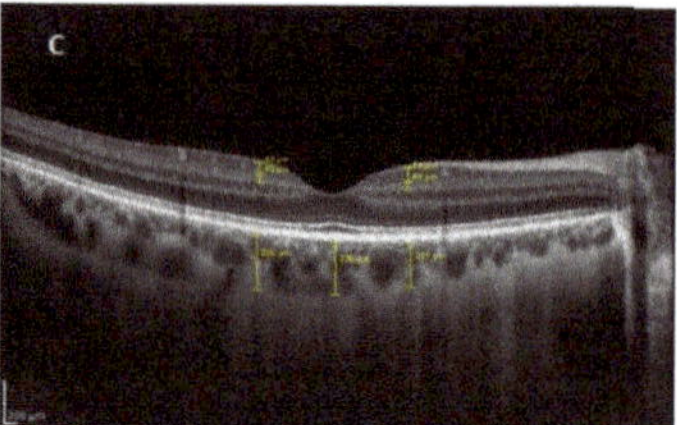

Figure 2. Ganglion cell layer, inner plexiform layer and choroidal thickness measurements. (**A**). Scanning laser ophthalmoscopy image of the macula. Green line is showing the cross-section of a optic coherence tomography (OCT) B-scan like in B and C. (**B**). OCT B-scan of a patient with primary insomnia. (**C**). OCT B-scan of a healthy control. *: Ganglion cell layer, ¥: Inner plexiform layer, †: Choroid.

2.2. Clinical Measurments

Insomnia severity index (ISI) quick inventory: The ISI is a seven-item questionnaire measuring insomnia symptoms and their impact on daytime functioning [26]. Scores range from 0–7 as no insomnia, 8–14 as sub-threshold, 15–21 as moderate, and 22–28 as severe insomnia.

Pittsburgh sleep quality index (PSQI): The Pittsburgh sleep quality index (PSQI) [27] was developed to evaluate the subjective sleep quality over the past month. PSQI composed of a total of twenty-four items, although the quality of sleep is calculated only by nineteen items that are self-rated. The seven-component scores range from 0 to 21 in total; higher scores indicate worse sleep quality.

2.3. Statistical Analysis

Demographic and clinical data of the participants were analyzed by descriptive statistics. Student *t*-tests were conducted to compare groups on continuous variables and chi-square analyses were used to compare groups on categorical variables. Data were checked whether they were normally distributed, and all relevant statistical analysis were conducted accordingly. For group comparisons on the OCT measurements, post-hoc corrections for multiple comparisons were not done due to the exploratory nature of the study. Spearman correlations were performed to analyze the relationship between the clinical variables of sleep and OCT parameters in the patient with primary insomnia and HC separately. Multiple stepwise regression analyses were conducted for each dependent variables and selection continued until all of the variables were either included or excluded. The predictor variables were stated each of the OCT measurements (as depended variables). All analyses were performed using IBM SPSS for Mac, Version 22.0 and statistical significance was set at a *p*-value of 0.05.

3. Results

3.1. Sample Characteristics

The demographic and clinical variables of the participants is shown in Table 1. The groups did not differ from each other in terms of age, gender, and BMI. According to the specified cut off scores of the ISI, 30 (26.1%) of the participants were suffering from a mild, 31 (27.0%) from a moderate, and 18 (15.7%) from a severe insomnia (Table 1).

Table 1. Demographic and clinical characteristics of the studied population.

	Insomnia $N = 52$	Healthy Controls $N = 45$	χ^2 (df)/t (df)	p Value
Age (mean ± SD)	43.0 ± 11.7	40.3 ± 12.2	1.125 (91.7)	0.26
Gender (female, number)	40	31	0.794 (1)	0.49
BMI	26.7 ± 5.8	27.6 ± 5.8	−0.780 (92.3)	0.43
Smoking (yes, number)	16	21	0.270 (1)	0.66
PSQI (mean ± SD)	12.3 ± 3.3	4.3 ± 2.0	14.436 (85.4)	<0.001
ISI (mean ± SD)	19.9 ± 4.2	5.7 ± 2.1	−21.577	<0.001
Duration of the insomnia (month, mean ± SD)	31.6 ± 45.2			

BMI, body-mass index; PSQI, Pittsburgh sleep quality index; ISI, insomnia severity index. Sociodemographic variables were calculated by Chi-square tests for categorical variables and *t*-test for continuous variables. The significance threshold was set at 0.05.

3.2. Group Comparisons according to the Optical Coherence Tomography Results

There were statistically significant differences between the patients with primary insomnia and the healthy control in terms of the RNFL-G ($z = -2.260$, $p = 0.024$) and RNFL-NI ($z = -2.591$, $p = 0.010$) measurement. All areas of RNFL measurement are presented in Table 2.

Table 2. Comparisons RNFL variables between patients with primary insomnia and healthy controls.

	Insomnia $N = 52$	Healthy Controls $N = 45$	z/t	p Value
RNFL-G (mean ± SD)	101.32 ± 9.12	105.48 ± 7.81	$z = -2.260$	0.024 *
RNFL-T (mean ± SD)	73.53 ± 12.35	76.53 ± 12.41	$z = -1.299$	0.194
RNFL-TS (mean ± SD)	140.94 ± 19.69	141.71 ± 19.01	$z = -0.416$	0.677
RNFL-TI (mean ± SD)	144.19 ± 26.93	139.28 ± 29.98	$z = -0.651$	0.515
RNFL-N (mean ± SD)	77.53 ± 12.88	78.35 ± 14.58	$z = -0.916$	0.360
RNFL-NS (mean ± SD)	122.28 ± 25.13	117.06 ± 25.13	$t = 1.062$	0.288
RNFL-NI (mean ± SD)	109.76 ± 21.84	118.84 ± 25.64	$z = -2.591$	0.010 *

RNFL, retinal nerve fiber layer; TS, temporal superior; TI, temporal inferior; NS, nasal superior; NI, nasal inferior. *, The significant threshold 0.05.

There were statistically significant differences between the patients with primary insomnia and the healthy control in terms of the IPL-N (38.69 ± 4.36 vs. 43.51 ± 4.58; $t = -5.282$, $p < 0.001$) and IPL-T (37.40 ± 5.54 vs. 42.82 ± 5.36; $t = -4.880$, $p < 0.001$) measurement. There were no statistically significant differences between the patients with primary insomnia and the healthy control in terms of the GCL-N (52.42 ± 6.92 vs. 50.68 ± 6.29; $t = -5.282$, $p = 0.20$) and GCL-T (45.84 ± 8.02 vs. 43.04 ± 6.92; $t = -4.880$, $p = 0.068$). Comparisons of GCL and IPL measurements are presented in Figure 3.

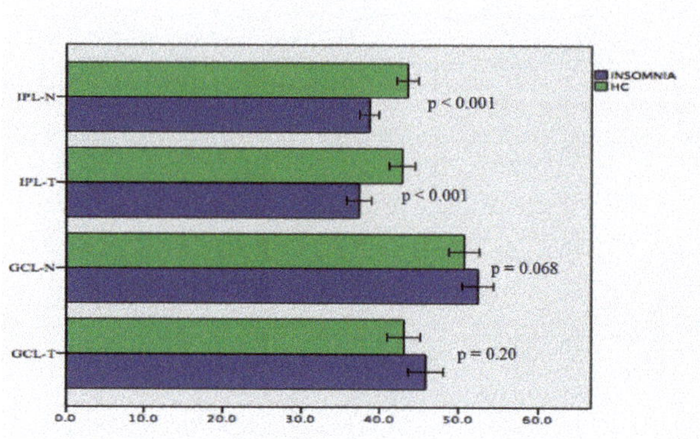

Figure 3. Comparisons of GCL and IPL between patients with primary insomnia and healthy controls. Abbreviations: IPL-N, inner plexiform layer- nasal; IPL-T, inner plexiform layer-temporal; GCL-N, ganglion cell layer-nasal; GCL-T, ganglion cell layer-temporal; HC, healthy controls.

The patients with primary insomnia and healthy controls differed statistically significant from each other in terms of all choroidal measurements (Figure 4).

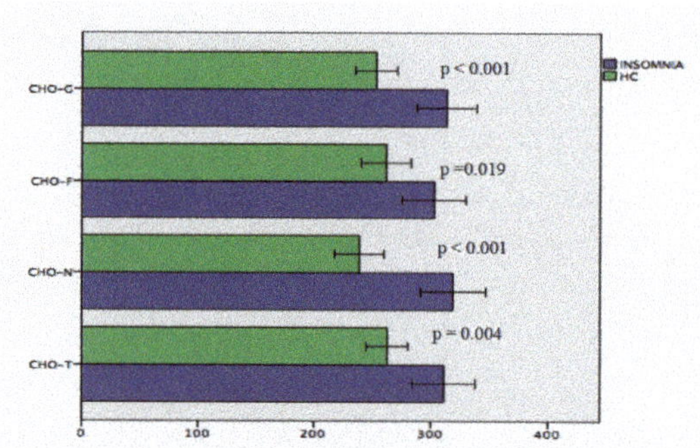

Figure 4. Comparisons of CHO-N (319.28 ± 100.01 vs. 238.95 ± 69.92); CHO-T (311.38 ± 97.34 vs. 262.75 ± 58.91); CHO-F (302.90 ± 98.48 vs. 261.66 ± 70.32); CHO-G (313.65 ± 92.46 vs. 253.21 ± 58.87) between patients with primary insomnia and healthy controls.

3.3. Correlation of the Clinical Variables with the Optical Coherence Tomography Measurements

Spearman correlation analyses were conducted between the clinical variables (ISI, PSQI, MEQ, BMI, duration of the insomnia) and the measurements of OCT in the patients with primary insomnia. The results revealed that the ISI score was correlated with RNFL-NI (Rho= −0.328, $p = 0.020$) and RNFL-G (Rho= −0.306, $p = 0.031$). The duration of the insomnia and BMI were not found correlated with any parameter. No significant correlation was found in the HC.

3.4. Stepwise Linear Regression Results

To examine the unique associations between the clinical variables, i.e., age, sex, BMI, PSQI, ISI, and OCT variables a stepwise linear regression analysis using the backward method was performed. The dependent variables were each of the OCT measurements. No variables were entered into the equation with the thicknesses of RNFL-TS, RNFL-T, RNFL-N, RNFL-NS, Macula, IPL-T, and GCL-T in patients with primary insomnia. Table 3 reports summary of the predictors of the stepwise linear regression analyses for the thickness of RNFL-G, RNFL-NI, RNFL-TI, GCL-N, IPL-N, CHO-G, CHO-N, and CHO-T. (Table 3).

Table 3. Summary of multiple regression analysis with the OCT parameters in patients with primary insomnia ($n = 52$).

Dependent Variable	Predictor/s	B	SE	β	t	p
CHO-G	Age	−3.806	1.088	−0.451	−3.497	0.001
CHO-T	Age	−3.811	1.022	−0.474	−3.727	0.001
CHO-N	Age	−4.421	0.923	−0.566	−4.731	<0.001
	ISI	−218.185	100.660	−0.260	−2.168	0.035
CHO-F	Age	−4.256	1.047	−0.506	−4.065	<0.001
RNFL-G	ISI	−25.422	11.419	−0.306	−2.226	0.031
RNFL-NI	ISI	−64.947	27.003	−0.328	−2.405	0.020
RNFL-TI	Gender	27.623	8.230	0.436	3.356	0.002
IPL-N	Gender	3.303	1.392	0.324	2.373	0.022

B = unstandardized beta coefficient; SE = standard error; β = standardized beta coefficient. CHO-N, choroid nasal; CHO-T, choroid temporal; CHO-F, choroid fovea; CHO-G, choroid global; RNFL, retinal nerve fiber layer; TI, temporal inferior; NI, nasal inferior; IPL-N, inner plexiform layer- nasal; GCL-N, ganglion cell layer-nasal; ISI, insomnia severity index.

4. Discussion

The major findings of this study were that patients with primary insomnia had the thinning of RNFL-G, RNFL-NI, and IPL-T, IPL-N thicknesses compared to healthy controls; the thinning of RNFL- G and RNFL-NI were correlated with the severity of insomnia. Second, our results showed the significant thickening of CHO-G, CHO-T, CHO-N, and CHO-F in patients with primary insomnia compared to healthy controls; and regression analyses indicated the ISI score as a predictor for the thickness of RNFL-NI and CHO-N in patients with primary insomnia.

Regarding our results, the global retinal nerve fiber layer thinning in patients with insomnia might be an effect of neurodegeneration or neurochemical dysregulation. Insomnia is associated with reduced brain activation, blood flow, or glucose metabolism. There is a growing body of evidence that sleep disruption may also accelerate the progression of pathology of neurodegenerative diseases via defective mitochondrial dynamics and axonal transport [28]. The RNFL is found more sensitive to vascular changes associated with gliosis and inflammation than other layers of the retina, which would influence OCT measurements [29]. Also, the RNFL is first-order neurons, with the unmyelinated ganglion cell axons that project to the lateral geniculate nucleus of the thalamus, it provides sensory input to the visual cortex, and the thinning of the retinal nerve fiber layer following by lesions of the thalamic-visual pathway in humans is hypothesized as retrograde trans-synaptic axonal degeneration (RTSD) [30,31] and identified by optical coherence tomography [31]. The thalamus is also a major region involved in the pathophysiology of insomnia, sleep-wake rhythms and hyperarousal [32]. Previous studies have reported functional and structural abnormalities in the thalamus in patients with insomnia [33,34]. The disrupted white-matter integrity of thalamus [35], the reduced bilateral thalamic grey-matter volume after sleep deprivation [33], atrophic changes [36], and the structural and metabolic alterations in the thalamus have been replicated in neuroimaging studies [35] in patients with insomnia. Therefore, RTSD may lead to the thinning of RNFL due to the effect of the thalamocortical dysfunction by insomnia [37].

We found also the nasal sector (nasal inferior) of RNFL was significantly affected in our patients. The segmentation analysis of the retinal layers might add important information about changes in the different retinal regions since the global thickness of RNFL alone may not reflect the pathophysiology of diseases [38,39]. Retinal ganglion cell axons are distributed in a specific topographic manner at the optic nerve head and the axons from the nasal and temporal segments of the retina have different anatomical microenvironments that might change the neurodegenerative pattern [40]. Many neurodegenerative disorders have been characterized by the different pattern of RGCL loss, and optic nerve degeneration [38]. For example, multiple system atrophy displays an OCT pattern more similar to Alzheimer whereas the OCT pattern of Huntington is closer to Parkinson's disease [38]. Also, the relative sparing of the RNFL was found predominantly in the temporal quadrant in patients with PD, and in the superior and inferior RNFL quadrants in patients with AZ [35]. According to a meta-analysis, there was significant with a moderate effect size thinning of the RNFL for the global and nasal region in the patients with SZ and BD [14]. Another study found significant thinning of the nasal parafoveal RNFL in SZ compared to HC, but not in the overall or temporal region [41]. Our findings are more similar to the results of the study with the patients with SZ and BD in terms of the location of thinning of the RNFL in the global and nasal region. Although sleep disorders are seen commonly in both schizophrenia and bipolar disorder, it is difficult to interpret our data; global thinning of RNFL and the specific distribution of nasal inferior RNFL requires replication in independent samples with insomnia.

We found the thinning of IPL-T and IPL-N in patients with primary insomnia compared to HC. The retinal ganglion cell and inner nuclear layers of the retina contain functionally autonomous circadian clocks [6]. Also, dopaminergic (DA) amacrines and ganglion neurons of retina express key elements of the circadian autoregulatory gene network with the highest proportion in DA neurons (30%) and amacrine cells are inhibitory interneurons and with bipolar cells extend presynaptic dendrites to the IPL where they synapse with retinal ganglion cells [42]. Furthermore, almost all dopaminergic amacrine cells are GABAergic and are located at the boundary of inner nuclear layer (INL) and IPL and branched in S1 lamina of the IPL. Primary insomnia suggested as a hyperarousal state of the CNS and the consistent findings of proton magnetic resonance spectroscopy showed that insomnia is associated with lower GABA levels in the parieto-occipital cortex [43,44] and anterior cingulate [45] by reflecting presynaptic concentrations of GABA [46]. Therefore, our findings might reflect the effect of decreased level of GABA; and are in line with the studies that showed the dysregulation of melatonin and dopamine levels which might cause the thinning of IPL. RTSD might be also one of another cause of the atrophy of the inner retinal layers, such as the GCL and IPL. Therefore, researchers suggested that the decreases in GCL and IPL may reflect neuronal atrophy, synaptic loss and have shown that IPL measurements might be better biomarkers of symptom severity than the RNFL in patients with multiple sclerosis [47].

We found the thickening of choroidal layers (CHO-Global, Temporal, Nasal, and Foveal) statistically significant in patients with primary insomnia compared than healthy controls, and the regression analyses indicated that the age and severity of insomnia score were predictors for the thickness of CHO-Nasal in patients with primary insomnia. The choroid is likewise well established in humans to show significant diurnal alterations in thickness, and daily rhythms of light exposure are determined to perform a pivotal role in the synchronization of these circadian rhythms [48]. One of the potential mechanisms is that the light-induced increase of retinal DA [49] results in nitric oxide (NO) release and NO leads to an increase of choroidal blood flow and density [50]. Furthermore, this process is plausible in the literature and affects the choroidal bloodstream variations in feedback to shifting light conditions [50]. Previous investigators have demonstrated that the choroid has a relative peak thickness early in the morning and progressive decrease during the day to a relative nadir at 5:00 PM [50]. In our study, measurements of all individuals were performed between 8.00–10.00 in the morning. Therefore, we can assume that insomnia leads to choroidal thickness if we do not consider the measurement time as a confounding factor. Moreover, we found that the severity of insomnia is a predictor for the choroidal thickness. Insomnia is a clinical condition that affects circadian rhythm disruption and the proportion of exposure to the daylight. So the above-mentioned retinal dopamine and nitric oxide-mediated vascular responses caused by light responses may change the thickness of choroid.

There are several limitations to our study. The cross-sectional nature of the study does not allow us to explore the causal relationships between insomnia and retinal changes. We did not study with objective parameters in sleep. Therefore, future investigations should examine both subjective and objective parameters of sleep. Also, using actigraphy should be considered for having high concordance with polysomnography in healthy adults. We included the patients in the study from a single outpatient clinic, and our patients were mostly women. Therefore, a multi-center and homogeneity in gender studies are required to test better our results.

5. Conclusions

The inner retinal layers have been demonstrated in many disorders as a biomarker of the neurodegeneration, but the confounding factors may reveal that these findings have not been fully recognized yet. This OCT study is the first to show a significant decrease of the retinal nerve fiber and inner plexiform layers in patients with primary insomnia versus healthy controls. Our explorative data might provide a rationale for further examination of insomnia as a potential confounder factor for the OCT findings in patients with ocular and non-ocular diseases. Likewise, our study indicated that the thickness of choroid can show a statistically significant increase in patients with primary insomnia and may have implications to understand the impact of sleep upon the pathogenesis of retinal physiology.

Author Contributions: Conceptualization, C.S.; methodology, C.S., A.E., M.O., H.O.; software, C.S., A.E.; validation, C.S., A.E., and H.O.; formal analysis, C.S.; investigation, C.S., M.O.; resources, C.S. and H.O.; data curation, C.S.; writing—original draft preparation, C.S., M.O., A.E., H.O.; writing—review and editing, C.S.; visualization, C.S.; supervision, H.O.; project administration, C.S., H.O. All authors have read and agreed to the published version of the manuscript.

Conflicts of Interest: The authors declare no conflict of interest.

References

1. Riemann, D.; Nissen, C.; Palagini, L.; Otte, A.; Perlis, M.L.; Spiegelhalder, K. The neurobiology, investigation, and treatment of chronic insomnia. *Lancet. Neurol.* **2015**, *14*, 547–558. [CrossRef]
2. Ohayon, M.M. Epidemiology of insomnia: What we know and what we still need to learn. *Sleep Med. Rev.* **2002**, *6*, 97–111. [CrossRef] [PubMed]
3. Fernandez-Mendoza, J.; Vgontzas, A.N. Insomnia and its impact on physical and mental health. *Curr. Psychiatry Rep.* **2013**, *15*, 418. [CrossRef] [PubMed]
4. Chu, E.M.; Kolappan, M.; Barnes, T.R.E.; Joyce, E.M.; Ron, M.A. A window into the brain: An in vivo study of the retina in schizophrenia using optical coherence tomography. *Psychiatry Res.* **2012**, *203*, 89–94. [CrossRef] [PubMed]
5. Appaji, A. Retinal vascular tortuosity in schizophrenia and bipolar disorder. *Schizophr. Res.* **2019**, *212*, 26–32. [CrossRef] [PubMed]
6. Ko, G.Y. Circadian regulation in the retina: From molecules to network. *Eur. J. Neurosci.* **2018**, *51*, 194–216. [CrossRef]
7. Ruan, G.X.; Zhang, D.Q.; Zhou, T.; Yamazaki, S.; McMahon, D.G. Circadian organization of the mammalian retina. *Proc. Natl. Acad. Sci. USA* **2006**, *103*, 9703–9708. [CrossRef]
8. DeVera, C.; Baba, K.; Tosini, G. Retinal Circadian Clocks are Major Players in the Modulation of Retinal Functions and Photoreceptor Viability. *Yale J. Biol. Med.* **2019**, *92*, 233–240.
9. McMahon, D.G.; Iuvone, P.M.; Tosini, G. Circadian organization of the mammalian retina: From gene regulation to physiology and diseases. *Prog. Retin. Eye Res.* **2014**, *39*, 58–76. [CrossRef]
10. Mukherjee, C.; Al-Fahad, Q.; Elsherbiny, S. The role of optical coherence tomography in therapeutics and conditions, which primarily have systemic manifestations: A narrative review. *Ther. Adv. Ophthalmol.* **2019**, *11*, 2515841419831155. [CrossRef]

11. Gordon-Lipkin, E.; Chodkowski, B.; Reich, D.S.; Smith, S.A.; Pulicken, M.; Balcer, L.J.; Frohman, E.M.; Cutter, G.; Calabresi, P.A. Retinal nerve fiber layer is associated with brain atrophy in multiple sclerosis. *Neurology* **2007**, *69*, 1603–1609. [CrossRef] [PubMed]

12. Grazioli, E.; Zivadinov, R.; Weinstock-Guttman, B.; Lincoff, N.; Baier, M.; Wong, J.R.; Hussein, S.; Cox, J.L.; Hojnacki, D.; Ramanathan, M. Retinal nerve fiber layer thickness is associated with brain MRI outcomes in multiple sclerosis. *J. Neurol. Sci.* **2008**, *268*, 12–17. [CrossRef] [PubMed]

13. Silverstein, S.M.; Paterno, D.; Cherneski, L.; Green, S. Optical coherence tomography indices of structural retinal pathology in schizophrenia. *Psychol. Med.* **2018**, *48*, 2023–2033. [CrossRef] [PubMed]

14. Lizano, P.; Bannai, D.; Lutz, O.; Kim, L.A.; Miller, J.; Keshavan, M. A Meta-analysis of Retinal Cytoarchitectural Abnormalities in Schizophrenia and Bipolar Disorder. *Schizophr. Bull.* **2019**, *46*, 43–53. [CrossRef]

15. Yildiz, M.; Alim, S.; Batmaz, S.; Demir, S.; Songur, E.; Ortak, H.; Demirci, K. Duration of the depressive episode is correlated with ganglion cell inner plexifrom layer and nasal retinal fiber layer thicknesses: Optical coherence tomography findings in major depression. *Psychiatry Res. Neuroimaging* **2016**, *251*, 60–66. [CrossRef]

16. Moschos, M.M.; Gonidakis, F.; Varsou, E.; Markopoulos, I.; Rouvas, A.; Ladas, I.; Papadimitriou, G.N. Anatomical and functional impairment of the retina and optic nerve in patients with anorexia nervosa without vision loss. *Br. J. Ophthalmol.* **2011**, *95*, 1128–1133. [CrossRef]

17. Palagini, L.; Bastien, C.H.; Marazziti, D.; Ellis, J.G.; Riemann, D. The key role of insomnia and sleep loss in the dysregulation of multiple systems involved in mood disorders: A proposed model. *J. Sleep Res.* **2019**, *28*, e12841. [CrossRef]

18. Logan, R.W.; McClung, C.A. Rhythms of life: Circadian disruption and brain disorders across the lifespan. *Nat. Rev. Neurosci.* **2019**, *20*, 49–65. [CrossRef]

19. Katz, D.A.; McHorney, C.A. Clinical correlates of insomnia in patients with chronic illness. *Arch. Int. Med.* **1998**, *158*, 1099–1107. [CrossRef]

20. Lane, J.M.; Jones, S.E.; Dashti, H.S.; Wood, A.R.; Aragam, K.G.; van Hees, V.T.; Strand, L.B.; Winsvold, B.S.; Wang, H.; Bowden, J.; et al. Biological and clinical insights from genetics of insomnia symptoms. *Nat. Genet.* **2019**, *51*, 387–393. [CrossRef]

21. Gracitelli, C.P.; Duque-Chica, G.L.; Roizenblatt, M.; Moura, A.L.; Nagy, B.V.; de Ragot, M.G.; Borba, P.D.; Teixeira, S.H.; Tufik, S.; Ventura, D.F.; et al. Intrinsically photosensitive retinal ganglion cell activity is associated with decreased sleep quality in patients with glaucoma. *Ophthalmology* **2015**, *122*, 1139–1148. [CrossRef] [PubMed]

22. Wu, C.Y.; Riangwiwat, T.; Rattanawong, P.; Nesmith, B.L.W.; Deobhakta, A. Association Of Obstructive Sleep Apnea With Central Serous Chorioretinopathy And Choroidal Thickness: A Systematic Review and Meta-Analysis. *Retina* **2018**, *38*, 1642–1651. [CrossRef] [PubMed]

23. Schaal, S.; Sherman, M.P.; Nesmith, B.; Barak, Y. Untreated Obstructive Sleep Apnea Hinders Response to Bevacizumab in Age-Related Macular Degeneration. *Retina* **2016**, *36*, 791–797. [CrossRef] [PubMed]

24. Xin, C.; Wang, J.; Zhang, W.; Lang, L.; Peng, X. Retinal and choroidal thickness evaluation by SD-OCT in adults with obstructive sleep apnea-hypopnea syndrome (OSAS). *Eye* **2014**, *28*, 415–421. [CrossRef]

25. Bastien, C.H.; Vallieres, A.; Morin, C.M. Validation of the Insomnia Severity Index as an outcome measure for insomnia research. *Sleep Med.* **2001**, *2*, 297–307. [CrossRef]

26. Buysse, D.J.; Reynolds, C.F., III; Monk, T.H.; Berman, S.R.; Kupfer, D.J. The Pittsburgh Sleep Quality Index: A new instrument for psychiatric practice and research. *Psychiatry Res.* **1989**, *28*, 193–213. [CrossRef]

27. Malhotra, R.K. Neurodegenerative Disorders and Sleep. *Sleep Med. Clin.* **2018**, *13*, 63–70. [CrossRef]

28. Ortuno-Lizaran, I.; Esquiva, G.; Beach, T.G.; Serrano, G.E.; Adler, C.H.; Lax, P.; Cuenca, N. Degeneration of human photosensitive retinal ganglion cells may explain sleep and circadian rhythms disorders in Parkinson's disease. *Acta Neuropathol. Commun.* **2018**, *6*, 90. [CrossRef]

29. Dinkin, M. Trans-synaptic Retrograde Degeneration in the Human Visual System: Slow, Silent, and Real. *Curr. Neurol. Neurosci. Rep.* **2017**, *17*, 16. [CrossRef]

30. Jindahra, P.; Petrie, A.; Plant, G.T. Retrograde trans-synaptic retinal ganglion cell loss identified by optical coherence tomography. *Brain* **2009**, *132 (Pt 3)*, 628–634. [CrossRef]

31. Lugaresi, E. The thalamus and insomnia. *Neurology* **1992**, *42 (Suppl. S6)*, 28–33.

32. Liu, C.; Kong, X.Z.; Liu, X.; Zhou, R.; Wu, B. Long-term total sleep deprivation reduces thalamic gray matter volume in healthy men. *Neuroreport* **2014**, *25*, 320–323. [CrossRef] [PubMed]

33. Spiegelhalder, K.; Regen, W.; Baglioni, C.; Riemann, D.; Winkelman, J.W. Neuroimaging studies in insomnia. *Curr. Psychiatry Rep.* **2013**, *15*, 405. [CrossRef] [PubMed]

34. Kang, J.M.K.; Joo, S.W.; Son, Y.; Kim, H.K.; Ko, K.; Lee, J.S.; Kang, S. Low white-matter integrity between the left thalamus and inferior frontal gyrus in patients with insomnia disorder. *J. Psychiatry Neurosci.* **2018**, *43*, 366–374. [CrossRef] [PubMed]

35. Koo, D.L.; Shin, J.H.; Lim, J.S.; Seong, J.K.; Joo, E.Y. Changes in subcortical shape and cognitive function in patients with chronic insomnia. *Sleep Med.* **2017**, *35*, 23–26. [CrossRef]

36. Usrey, W.M.; Alitto, H.J. Visual Functions of the Thalamus. *Annu. Rev. Vis. Sci.* **2015**, *1*, 351–371. [CrossRef]

37. La Morgia, C.; Di Vito, L.; Carelli, V.; Carbonelli, M. Patterns of Retinal Ganglion Cell Damage in Neurodegenerative Disorders: Parvocellular vs Magnocellular Degeneration in Optical Coherence Tomography Studies. *Front. Neurol.* **2017**, *8*, 710. [CrossRef]

38. Polo, V.; Satue, M.; Gavin, A.; Vilades, E.; Orduna, E.; Cipres, M.; Garcia-Campayo, J.; Navarro-Gil, M.; Larrosa, J.M. Ability of swept source OCT to detect retinal changes in patients with bipolar disorder. *Eye* **2019**, *33*, 549–556. [CrossRef]

39. Hogan, M.J.; Alvarado, J.A.; Weddell, J.E. *Histology of the Human Eye*; An atlas and textbook; Saunders: Philadelphia, PA, USA, 1971.

40. Samani, N.N.; Proudlock, F.A.; Siram, V.; Suraweera, C.; Hutchinson, C.; Nelson, C.P.; Al-Uzri, M.; Gottlob, I. Retinal Layer Abnormalities as Biomarkers of Schizophrenia. *Schizophr. Bull.* **2018**, *44*, 876–885. [CrossRef]

41. Balasubramanian, R.; Gan, L. Development of Retinal Amacrine Cells and Their Dendritic Stratification. *Curr. Ophthalmol. Rep.* **2014**, *2*, 100–106. [CrossRef]

42. Morgan, P.T.; Pace-Schott, E.F.; Mason, G.F.; Forselius, E.; Fasula, M.; Valentine, G.W.; Sanacora, G. Cortical GABA levels in primary insomnia. *Sleep* **2012**, *35*, 807–814. [CrossRef] [PubMed]

43. Winkelman, J.W.; Buxton, O.M.; Jensen, J.E.; Benson, K.L.; O'Connor, S.P.; Wang, W.; Renshaw, P.F. Reduced brain GABA in primary insomnia: Preliminary data from 4T proton magnetic resonance spectroscopy (1H-MRS). *Sleep* **2008**, *31*, 1499–1506. [CrossRef] [PubMed]

44. Plante, D.T.; Jensen, J.E.; Schoerning, L.; Winkelman, J.W. Reduced gamma-aminobutyric acid in occipital and anterior cingulate cortices in primary insomnia: A link to major depressive disorder? *Neuropsychopharmacology* **2012**, *37*, 1548–1557. [CrossRef]

45. Kay, D.B.; Buysse, D.J. Hyperarousal and Beyond: New Insights to the Pathophysiology of Insomnia Disorder through Functional Neuroimaging Studies. *Brain Sci.* **2017**, *7*, 23. [CrossRef] [PubMed]

46. Saidha, S.; Syc, S.B.; Durbin, M.K.; Eckkstein, C.; Oakley, J.D.; Meyer, S.A.; Conger, A.; Frohman, T.C.; Newsome, S.; Ratchford, J.N.; et al. Visual dysfunction in multiple sclerosis correlates better with optical coherence tomography derived estimates of macular ganglion cell layer thickness than peripapillary retinal nerve fiber layer thickness. *Mult. Scler. J.* **2011**, *17*, 1449–1463. [CrossRef]

47. Tan, C.S.; Ouyang, Y.; Ruiz, H.; Sadda, S.R. Diurnal variation of choroidal thickness in normal, healthy subjects measured by spectral domain optical coherence tomography. *Investig. Ophthalmol. Vis. Sci.* **2012**, *53*, 261–266. [CrossRef]

48. Brainard, G.C.; Morgan, W.W. Light-induced stimulation of retinal dopamine: A dose-response relationship. *Brain Res.* **1987**, *424*, 199–203. [CrossRef]

49. Huemer, K.H.; Garhofer, G.; Aggermann, T.; Kolodjascna, J.; Schmetterer, L.; Fuchsjager-Mayrl, G. Role of nitric oxide in choroidal blood flow regulation during light/dark transitions. *Investig. Ophthalmol. Vis. Sci.* **2007**, *48*, 4215–4219. [CrossRef]

50. Read, S.A.; Pieterse, E.C.; Alanso-Caneiro, D.; Bormann, R.; Hong, S.; Lo, C.; Richer, R.; Syed, A.; Tran, L. Daily morning light therapy is associated with an increase in choroidal thickness in healthy young adults. *Sci. Rep.* **2018**, *8*, 8200. [CrossRef]

MDPI

St. Alban-Anlage 66

4052 Basel

Switzerland

Tel. +41 61 683 77 34

Fax +41 61 302 89 18

www.mdpi.com

Brain Sciences Editorial Office

E-mail: brainsci@mdpi.com

www.mdpi.com/journal/brainsci